Plunge into Darkness

A Fighter's Fight with Cancer

By Dave & Barbie Renfroe

PLUNGE INTO DARKNESS
A FIGHTER'S FIGHT WITH CANCER

Copyright Dave & Barbie Renfroe, 2018

ISBN 978-0-692-12221-1

Learn more online about Barbie's struggle at *davebarbierenfroe.com*

Cover design by Rob Bignell

Manufactured in the United States of America
First printing May 2018

ACKNOWLEDGEMENTS

I would like to thank our families who have stuck by us through the worst and the best.

All of those who have offered prayers over the years.

The doctors, nurses and countless medical professionals who have provided care with kindness and compassion.

All of my brothers and sisters at church.

My employers who have treated Barbie like family when she needed to tag along with me, and who understood when I needed to stay home with her.

Coworkers who have helped me carry on when I needed help.

A wonderful community and the neighbors who came alongside and helped pull the load.

Mr. Rob Bignell, the editor who helped me navigate strange waters to get this out to everyone.

Most of all I want to thank my Lord and Savior Jesus Christ for everything.

Contents

Chapter 1
A Couple in Love

We said our goodnights and went to bed. It was a normal night as we lay down; the suitcase was packed for the upcoming weeks work on the road. Our son was in bed in the next room awaiting the call for school the next morning. Our names are Dave and Barbie, and this would be the night that our lives changed forever.

As we lay in bed around 2 a.m., the bed began to shake, and an odd moan came from Barbie's side of the bed. I sprang from bed and turned on the light to find her shaking and incoherent her body gripped in the thralls of what I would find out later was a grand mal seizure. As the seizure stopped, she slowly returned, but not all the way. I helped her get dressed; it was clear that something was terribly wrong, for she was not there, but in the distance. As we got her dressed and woke our son, we quickly loaded up, and began the 25 minute race to the emergency room. With another seizure on the way, I remember asking our 12 year old son to check and see if she was still breathing. What a terrible thing to ask a kid; as soon as we arrived in the ER, another seizure gripped her. As she shook and convulsed uncontrollably, we looked on in disbelief. All sense of control and order had disappeared from our lives in an instant.

As the minutes turned into hours, I went from the ER room to the waiting room, watching my wife slip further and further away, all while trying to comfort our son. Family began to arrive, and soon we were huddled in the waiting room, waiting for the test results to come. The ER doctor arrived and asked to talk with me, and explained that the CAT scan of her brain indicated "something" was there; I stood dazed, as he explained that it appeared to be a brain tumor, and they were taking her for an MRI to get a better look.

As night gave way to morning and test results confirmed the ER doctor's diagnosis, the swelling in her brain continued to draw her farther away, by morning all she seemed to be able to communicate was her name and address. As I sat there in the dark looking at my wife lying in bed, not able to remember my name, or our sons, my thoughts began to drift to the past.

I grew up on a small farm in southern Ohio; my father and mother moved there the year I was born. It was there that I grew up with my older brother and sister. The farm was a wonderful place for a kid to grow up. Dad worked in a steel mill and farmed when he was not at work; as the years went by, he added a neighboring farm on each side of the original farm and our farm grew to just over 400 aces, about 100 acres of bottomland, about the same was wooded, and the rest pasture for the cattle that dad always loved. I grew up helping dad farm and like most young boys wanted to be just like him; I always said that I would be a farmer when I grew up. I hunted the woods and fished the ponds and the creek that ran through the farm. As I grew, so did the desire and the love of the outdoors. After a trip to California, where I stayed with my uncle and worked in a machine shop making break parts for Indy cars, and another to Tennessee, where I worked in small job shop running lathes and drill presses, I started farming in partnership with dad. We raised cattle, corn, hay, tobacco and several acres of sweet corn that we marketed roadside at the local towns.

I was living with my parents and farming when I was in my late twenties, and it was about that time that I ran into this pretty girl who would become the love of my life. She had just came out of a bad marriage and had a young son of about two years old. She had moved back to stay with her parents for a little while and rented a small place close by. She had grown up within five miles of the farm, but we had never met. We dated for about a year and a half, but I was head over heels in love long before that. She was a frequent visitor to the farm, often helping out with the various chores and jobs to be done. We seemed to have everything in common – she loved animals of any kind, the outdoors, and the country farm life in general. After a year and a half of dating, I asked her if she would be my wife, and she said yes. The ceremony was nothing fancy, a local justice of the peace, a couple of witnesses, then back home, up early the next morning to pull and market sweet corn. We were in the middle of the harvest, and it would not wait for things like honeymoons.

We spent a lot of time talking about our future and dreaming of what it would be like. We would farm for a living on the family farm, build a log cabin back on the hill away from everything, grow old together, and sit in rocking chairs on the porch. Like most young couples making plans, there was no thought given to health or other problems. We went on camping trips around the farm to get the feel of the different possible house sites; we were just going to build once, and wanted it to be in the right place. But for now we lived in a trailer that dad rented out on the farm; we remodeled it with the proceeds from our first tobacco crop. It was around that time that we signed a 25-year lease with dad and took the majority of the farming operation on ourselves; he kept half of the cattle and continued to help raise, feed and care for them. He was around and working on something always; that's just who he is.

Things were going great. We did not have a lot, but we had each other, were in love, and were doing what we wanted to be doing. Things went well for a few years. My sister and brother-in-law, who lived across the road, moved into town to be closer to their jobs, and we moved into their vacated house. We continued to go along as we had, expanding the farming operation to include more acres of our main cash crops. We worked hard, from daylight to dark most days, and we still never got everything done that needed to be done.

We started another small venture that was to become one of the joys of Barbie's life –we purchased a male and later a female Golden Retriever with the intention of raising puppies to sell. After a couple of years, we had our first litter, it went very well and was a good source of additional money, plus the added bonus of being able to play with a lot of puppies. Life was good, we were still very happy, and it was time to be saving for the dream home. We had our spot picked out and knew what we wanted to put there. We found three vintage log cabins that had been dismantled down in the hills of Kentucky and purchased them and brought them home to store in a shed until we could start the next step.

With our expanded operation came the need to hire some additional help on the farm. I would take part of the help and do one job, and Barbie would take part to do another. Many days, we also still had the pleasure of working together. We ran the farm this way for a couple of years, and things were good. Then as we were getting close to starting our cabin, we had one of those years that every farmer dreads, the small creek running through our property in untimely late and severe flood. It destroyed most of our crops, and what was not affected by the flood was affected by the wet weather. We did carry crop insurance, but the percentage paid covers your cost, so most profit is lost. So we had a tough year, but it happens. We had enough saved to get by and the insurance would let us plant next year's crop, so we lived that winter by "There's always next year."

Next year came, and we planted our crops with high hopes, but it was not to be again. Poor weather and crop disease combined to give us poor crops once more, this time with the savings depleted from last year's losses and the bills coming in. Barbie went to a local store and took a job to help make ends meet, she would work evenings, and I would watch our son when I got in from the field. It was a big help but not enough. We talked about it and decided that I would go look for a job as a machinist, a field that I had been trained in and worked years before, and she would come home and take care of the house and our boy, and manage any workers we had to hire to harvest our crop.

With many mixed emotions late summer I started working second shift at a shop in town about 25 miles away. I work there through that winter, and as we planted the next year's crop, over that year we started to get back on track. We had to scale back on the crops a little since I could not be there full time. That year was OK, and as I went into the next winter at the shop, I was growing very discontented. I came home late every evening, Barbie would be in bed, she got up early when I was in bed, and we saw very little of each other in those days. This was not our dream. I told my co-workers that I would not be there in six months and they had a good laugh, saying you will be here just like the rest of us, to which I replied, "It won't be my back you're looking at in front of this lathe next year." I had no idea how I was going to make that happen, but I was intent on getting out of that shop.

I had also served as a field reporter for our local Farm Service Agency for several years; that position had me on neighboring farms measuring and appraising various crop, and it was there one day in the spring that the CED ask me the question, "Do you want to be a loss adjuster?"

To which I answered, "What is a loss adjuster? Never mind, what does it pay?"

He told me it was a contract position and would not be full-time but the pay rate was about 25 percent more than I was making at the time, so my thought was if I can work three quarters of the time, I can make the same and have more time to farm, so I said, "Sure sign me up."

To my surprise, two weeks later I had appointments for my first training, then the second, then I left the machine shop and embarked on a new career. I had six days of training on a very complex insurance program, a box full of manuals and forms, and I had no choice other than to learn it and make it work. I was assigned to an FSA office about three hours from home; when I walked in I was welcomed as the first loss adjuster they had seen and found 700 open claims. Soon afterwards, I was leaving home on Monday and coming back on Friday. I did not like being away, but with the combination of my per diem and mileage, we were getting caught up and closer to our dream.

During this time, Barbie was the farmer, running the whole operation in my absence. The first year in this position I worked almost full time, covering the entire state; the next year was much the same. I took my first contract with a private insurance company at that time and held two contracts; it appeared that I was a good fit for crop insurance. Barbie continued to keep things going on the farm, and I never failed to brag on her to the farmers I met while on the road. I would tell them how she kept everything running smooth while I was on the road, of how hard she worked in the fields, and how good all the crops looked. We were both very happy and relished our time together, and missed each other when I was on the road. I was sure that when things slowed that I would be home more, but for now this was just what we needed, we were getting closer to building our house. I eventually quit the position with the government as they phased out crop insurance. I then held contracts with always two and at one time three separate private crop insurance companies. I was home a little more by working multiple companies I got all the work closer to home from each company, so I could help out on the farm a little more, we had a pretty good crop, or maybe I should say Barbie did, and another in the field the next year.

Then came the day we had worked, hoped, and waited for – we got a dozer and excavator in to start preparing our house site. We had chosen a spot on the hill behind my dad's house; it was tucked into the edge of a small meadow with an old pond that had went dry, nestled into the corner of a woodlot that bordered a large meadow that we raised crops on and the pasture where cattle grazed, a wonderful view for growing old and sitting on the porch. We could see only one neighboring house when the leaves were off, but none when they were on. We repaired the old pond and dug our basement out. That spring and summer, we were torn between working on the road, farming and trying to get the house started. We decided to pour our basement using Styrofoam forms, finish it, move in then build the cabin on top, we wanted to do all we could out of pocket and not go into debt, as we already had witnessed what a bad year could do. We got our forms in and stored them in dad's garage and began working on the footer. We were able to complete it without too much problem, it was very hot and my dad while helping out had a heat stroke or something similar, which earned him a ride in the ambulance, but he recovered well. My father-in-law and I finished it, and we were ready for the next step, saving enough money to purchase the concrete and pay for the labor to pour the walls.

We were back on track, growing our crops and working for the crop insurance company, the summer was in full swing and the crops looked to be profitable. The sweet corn crop came and went, and the tobacco crop was topped and approaching harvest. I was home on a Sunday night, and the bags were packed to leave on Monday morning.

Chapter 2
Plunge into Darkness

As the longest night of my life gave way to morning, we consulted a neurosurgeon, who began administering medicine to reduce the swelling. As the swelling decreased, Barbie slowly started to return, but not all the way. She was almost childlike, not completely understanding what was going on but able to recognize everyone and to communicate again. As I continued to stare upon her with tear-filled eyes, time seemed to stand still, and after what seemed like an eternity, the long night began to give way to one of many very long days to come.

Some time during the night, I remember looking up and seeing my sister looking at me through the door, with tear-filled eyes she joined my long vigil until morning when our surgeon arrived and consulted with us. He explained that Barbie did have a brain tumor in the right frontal lobe of her brain, and that he would need to do surgery as soon as they could reduce the swelling. As he sat with us and explained all of the possible outcomes of the surgery, the possible losses of movement, short-term memory, speech, sight, along with the possibility of personality changes that ranged to severe to minor, and of course, death. As we sat through this very solemn conversation, Barbie sat with a smile on her face and listened intently, as I looked around the faces of our loved ones in the room, both our parents, my sister, myself, the doctor and Barbie, she was the only one who was smiling. After the doctor finished and asked if there were any question, Barbie looked and him and asked, "Are you going to cut my hair?"

It was then that it hit me like a bolt of lightning; I was going to have to make this life-changing decision for her; she had no idea that her life was in peril. She knew now that she was in the hospital and who everyone around her was, but the situation held no gravity for her. It would be up to me and the weight of that reality pressed on me like the weight of the world. The doctor had informed us that he wanted to operate first thing in the morning. I asked for some time alone with my wife to try to discuss the situation with her in hope of making her understand, in hope of some help in the life and death decision looming before me. We talked for some time, and I could tell it was not getting through; there was no fear, and no real understanding of the possible consequences, but she made a statement that seemed to indicate that she knew more than I thought, she simply said, "We have to do something; I can't stay this way." I was blown away by the straightforward, to the point, way that she stated this fact, the fact that made it clear what had to be done, I contacted the doctor and surgery was scheduled for 6 a.m. the next morning, the hardest decision of my life had been made, but having it behind me brought no relief, the weight pressing down on me only got heavier.

The long day gave way to yet another long night. As I sat beside her hospital bed I began to do something I had not done in earnest for many years; I fell on my knees and sought the Lord in prayer. I had been saved when I was 12 years old, and had attended church faithfully for five years after that. But as I grew older, I neglected my prayer life and the Bible, and the result was that when the temptations came around I was weak. I spent the next twenty years out of church living very much like the world around me. It was during this time that I met Barbie, we fell in love, and we got married. She had never been saved and only attended church a few times. So as the long night dragged on, I found myself going between prayer and drifting back into memories.

We had met about ten years earlier. Barbie was coming out of a difficult marriage and had a two-year-old son, she had moved back to the area where we had both grown up. Although she had grown up only a few miles away we had never met before, but through various friends our paths crossed, and we began to date. A year and a half later, we were married and she moved down to our family farm. For several years after that, we farmed for a living, raising tobacco, cattle, grain crops and produce, we were together always. We were blessed in that we hardly ever argued and we got along better than anyone we knew. I thought about the early mornings; we would get up before daylight and get breakfast and coffee, then go to our sweetcorn patch and start pulling corn, we would pull a truck load, get cleaned up and to town to sell it. On weekends, Barbie would take the first load while I pulled a second. I smiled thinking of the mornings eating raw sweet corn in the field for breakfast, or the strange looks our boy got sitting on the tailgate of the truck eating a raw ear of corn at the farmers market. I thought about the mornings spent side by side hoeing tobacco or one of the many other manual jobs involved in raising that crop. Life was good. It was hard, but we still had a great relationship, and we were very much in love and were determined to make it. I thought about the events that had led me to work in the shop, and how after about a year and a half of working in a local machine I walked into a job as a crop insurance adjuster, a job I really liked, but that came with no health insurance, but we were a couple of young healthy farmers, so it was not a big deal. At least that was what we thought at the time, but now it was. My mind reeled with the thoughts of the medical attention that she was going to be in need of; how was I going to be able to pay for it all? My thought went to the circumstances that led us to that point, the lost crops, the years we tried to get caught up the fact that we were both working off the farm to pay bills and still farming but still were not getting anywhere. We were trying to get a start in life and could not get any traction; little did we know that our whole perception of problems would change, we also did not know that the Lord was laying groundwork in our lives to help us later. We finally managed to save enough to start preparation on our house site, we bought forms for a poured wall basement and had the excavation completed around our house site, on the hill behind my parent's house, in a place where we could see no neighbors, just like we liked it. We poured the footer and were getting close to pouring the walls; this was a slow process as we would do a step as we got enough money, so the time span above was stretched across most of a year.

It was around this time that these things were going on that Barbie started getting headaches. We did not think anything was wrong, as we both spent a lot of time working out in the sun; we just thought it was no big thing, after all, we were a young and healthy couple working for our dreams.

As one might expect, the long night continued to wear on, sleep would not come to me, so I sat in the dark and watched her sleep, the *what will I do* thoughts and memories from the last ten years filling my mind. The things that I wished we had been able to do, places I would like for us to go, the thought one has in the dark by the beside of a loved one who may not make it. I thought about the days and trials that would follow, and how I was going to proceed. We had no health insurance and no savings to speak of; I considered how we would cope with what I was sure would be a long slow recovery after brain surgery. It sounded so scary, brain surgery. I knew that I would not be able to afford to hire anyone to take care of her while I worked, and to be honest did not want to be away from her to work. I spent much of the night regretting the time I had spent on the road working and away from home, and the decision was made – I would call my boss in the morning and let him know I would no longer be able to work for a time unknown. There was the matter of a living to be made, bills to be paid, and a crop in the field to be harvested, but none of that mattered anymore; there was only Barbie and what had to be done. Medical bills would pile up, with no income to pay them, not important, if I had to spend the rest of my life working and paying on bills, then so be it. The night continued to wear on, I alternated between worry, planning and praying sleep would not come, tears would not stop. I knew that Barbie had never been saved, and I knew what that would mean if she did not make it through the surgery, this weighed on me very heavy throughout the night, she would not be able to understand if I tried to explain, I sought the Lord and ask that she have another chance to make it right with Him. I had lived so far from him the past twenty years that I needed to be seeking him for myself, but I had only one concern on this night, and she lay sleeping in bed before me. I thought about our son, the young man spending the night with his grandparents, who would have school activities, first dates, first jobs, and what would hopefully be a wonderful life ahead of him. Would she be there to see it? I thought about what might lay before me, I played all the bad outcome through my mind and put myself through them as the night continued, I put myself through the suffering of each outcome just as if they had happened, thinking I was preparing myself, not realizing I was just bowering trouble from tomorrow, at that time, I had not yet tapped into the wisdom that belongs to us all:

Take therefore no thought for the morrow: for the morrow shall take thought for the things of itself. Sufficient unto the day is the evil thereof. (Mt 6:34)

It was absolutely true, I had plenty to worry about that day, and the last thing I needed to do was to borrow trouble from tomorrow; after all, I would have tomorrow to worry about those things, and it was getting close.

As the morning finally arrived, Barbie awoke, wondering what was going on. As we talked, the nurse came in with some medicine for her; taking it, she asked what it was for. The nurse explained that she was prepping her for surgery. "What surgery?" she asked. It dawned on me that all the events of the past day and two endless nights were not in Barbie's memory, the nurse, and I looked at each other, and I asked for a moment alone with my wife. I explained the situation to her, recounted the talk we had with the surgeon the day before, and told her that she was scheduled for surgery in a couple of hours. She looked at me and asked a very logical question – if I thought that we should get a second opinion and if we were rushing into this. The medicine had reduced her swelling enough that she was starting to think a little better, but it did not change the fact that she was in an emergency surgery situation. My sister worked at the hospital and had assured me that our surgeon had a great reputation and was very good. Now I found that I did not only have to make a life and death decision for her but would have to convince her that having the surgery was the best thing to do. Fortunately, our relationship was one of trust, so when I told her that it needed to be done and recounted some of the discussion we had with the doctor from the evening before, she said "OK." I asked the nurse back in, and they continued the preparations for surgery. I sat and wondered if I had done the right thing; all the doubts and fears I had when making the original decision came rushing back. It seemed that the time that had crawled by for so long began to fly by, and in no time my lovely wife was being wheeled out of our room and into pre-op. As our families gathered around, we stood and watched her go. Though surrounded by all my family, I had never felt so alone in my life. Fear rushed over me; all the questions and all the thoughts of every outcome that I had gone over in the long night before left my head spinning.

Chapter 3
Surgery

Just 28 hours after her seizure, my wife was being wheeled off to surgery. As I watched her go, tears filled my eyes, and fears filled my heart. This was not how our life is supposed to go, after all, she was just thirty four years old, we had only been married for eight years, and we were just getting started in life. It couldn't be over, could it?

After a while, the nurses got us to visit her in pre-op. When I walked in, I found her there awaiting her surgery, the front of her head shaved and IVs in her arms. I was struck with just how brave she was; to this day that is one of the bravest things I think I have ever witnessed. She would show me more courage in the weeks and months and years to come; her bravery and unrelenting fighting spirit would come to mark her fight. We all hugged her and told her of our love, and then the time came when we were told she was to be taken in. I was told the surgery would take about six hours. I did not want to let her go or say goodbye. I wondered if I would ever see her again, hear her laugh, see her smile. I said, "I love you and will see you in a little while." I hoped in my heart that would be the case.

Another long day was beginning. About thirty hours had passed since I had slept, and I had no desire to do so. As the minutes begin to tick off, each seemingly taking an hour each, we waited. I would make trips to the restroom and while I was there I would fall to my knees and pray, asking the Lord to bring her through this, praying that she would come through this with the mental capabilities to make the decision on where she would spend eternity, praying that the decision was not already made, asking for the strength to get through what lay before me, knowing that I did not possess that on my own.

As I returned to the waiting room, I am surrounded by our son, my parents, brother and sister and their spouses, Barbie's parents, brother and his wife, uncles and aunts from both sides, and our pastor and his wife. Every one made small talk, put on a brave front, tried to lighten the atmosphere but to no avail; the gravity of the situation weighed heavy on all. I would slip into thoughts and memories, thinking of my life before we had met, thinking how much better it had been since that day. I had spent many years in bars, pool halls, parties and anywhere else I thought that I could find a good time, having no real idea what a good time was. She had shown me just a few hours before that I had been one of the happiest men around.

We would occasionally get updates from the operating room. All was going as planned, as the hours dragged on. Loved ones took me to the cafeteria and tried to get me to eat something, but I could not get anything past the giant lump in my throat. Coffee would slide by, but that was about all. I don't know how many times I prayed that day, but I know it was more than I had altogether in the last several years. I could not imagine that as long as the last day and a half had been that is was only the first steps of a long decent into darkness that we were embarking on. I was in a fog, driven by emotions and sleeplessness; I was as drained as I have ever been. The sixth hour passed and no word. Family and

friends tried to comfort me. My brother and I spent time re-
membering hunts and fishing trips we had been on; my
brother and I have been constant companions in the woods
and local streams for many years, and I very comforted to
have him there. We talked about the good times. The family
all tried to remember the good times, tried to hide their tears
and their worry enough to ease mine, but attempts failed on
both fronts over and over again.

At last, the doctor emerged from the operating room and
led us into a consultation room; he explained that he had removed a tumor about the size of a golf ball from her right
frontal lobe, and that he had stopped short of clear borders.
He explained that he had stopped because the lab reports
had come back showing that it was a type of tumor that
would respond well to radiation treatments. Though he said
the report did not appear to him to be correct, he had no
choice but to follow the recommendations. He told us that
she had experienced another seizure while on the table, but
it was not a problem, and that he had woke her and all seemed to be ok. He told us that she had been taken to recovery
and that we could see her in about an hour. We all drew a
deep breath and allowed a short sigh of relief; she had survived the surgery, and at least the preliminary report was not
terrible.

Another attempt was made by family to get me to eat
something, and about a half of a cheeseburger made its way
past the lump, then it closed up tight, still thinking about
what my lovely wife had been through and what was sure to
come. As we sat at the table, my brother-in-law told me how
terrible I looked. I am sure he was right; I had jumped in the
first clothes I had found when I woke up, jeans, T-shirt, no
socks, tennis shoes, and a ball cap. That had been close to 40

high stress, sleepless hours earlier. He was probably being kind when using the explanative that he did, and no matter how bad I looked, I felt much worse. I still could not see any chance of the terrible pressure that I felt letting up.

When the time came that I was able to go into the ICU and visit, even though my sister had tried to prepare me for how she would look, I found my knees weak when I saw her. She had numerous machines hooked up to her, a drain coming from her bandaged head, IVs and leads. I was stunned; luckily, she had not yet awakened to see my reaction. I sat beside her bed as the parade of loved ones came through to see her, each looking on and trying to hide their reactions from me. As visiting hours came to an end, I prepared to go out into the waiting room but the nurse told me I was welcomed to stay and sit with her. As I sat and watched the monitors in the stillness and darkness of that terrifying room, each change sent fear through me. She had still not woke , and as I sat alone with her in the room, the anxiety built the quiet broken only by the strange sounds from the monitors, sounds that I did not understand. It all began to weigh on my nerves. I sat and watched her sleep, watched each move she made, jumped each time an unknown sound issued from the monitors. Finally, I could not take it any longer. I told the nurse I would be in the waiting room, and if there was any change to come and get me. When I returned, many of the visitors who had supported me through the longest day of my life began to go home; each hugged me and let me know they were there if needed. This is something we say lightly many times, but when meant like it was then it goes farther that can be expressed by mere words.

The long day faded into night. I did experience enough relief to finally get a meal down, and I was finally able to somewhat relax I went in and visited again when the next visiting hours came around, still no change, she still had not awoke, I sat and held her hand, talked to her, prayed by her bedside, the nurse assured me she was doing well, after a while I returned to the waiting room, now just me and her parents, around 10 o'clock I pulled three chairs together in the waiting room and laid down for the first time in roughly forty four hours, it did not take long to fall asleep, I slept the deep dreamless sleep of one who was exhausted, no tossing turning or in and out sleep, I was out.

I awoke to the sound of a nurse calling my name. Startled, I sat up, and fear rushed through my head. Had something happened, was there an emergency? There had to be or the nurse would not had come and woke me in the middle of the night. The nurse asked if I could come back for a minute. I immediately asked if Barbie was ok.

She said, "Well yes, as a matter of fact she may be doing a little too good."

Her response left me a little puzzled. I hurried back to her room to find Barbie sitting up in her bed, head wrapped, tubes sticking out, leads running from her to the monitors. She saw me and said, "Dave, when is that doctor coming?"

I was confused and asked her what she was talking about.

"It's two o'clock, and that doctor still has not shown up. If he is not here in ten minutes, we are leaving."

I could not help but smile. This sounded like my wife; often the task would be to keep her waiting on doctors when they are running late for an appointment. I explained to her that she had already had her surgery earlier that day, it was now the middle of the night, and she was doing fine. She had come through the surgery and was recovering.

She said in a tone of voice that expressed clearly that she

did not believe me, "Who told you that?"

I told her I had been there the whole day, that all of our family had been there, and we had waited as she went through her nearly seven-hour surgery. As the nurse walked by she said, "Nurse, have I had surgery?"

The nurse told her that she had, and all had went well.

She said, "Oh," laid back down with all of the frustration gone, closed her eyes, and went to sleep.

I returned to the waiting room, with an indescribable since of relief washing over me. We had talked, she had understood, she knew me, she acted like herself. I relayed the events to her parents, stretched out across my three chairs, and fell deeply back to sleep.

I awoke early the next morning and went in to visit. I found her awake, one side of her face swollen and discolored. She still had all of the awful tubes, wires and monitors hooked to her, but she was aware of her surroundings and knew what had happened and felt pretty good considering all that she had been through. As we sat and talked, I thought that maybe we had made it through, she had survived surgery, and appeared to be OK, maybe not completely herself but alive and on her way. Well, I was very relieved. As the family started coming in, I left for the first time in more than two days. I went to an aunt's house who lived close by, showered, and put on clean clothes that had been brought to me, had a homecooked breakfast, and went back to the hospital. I resisted all efforts to convince me lay down and get some sleep; it did not matter that several family members were with her, I was not, and that was unacceptable. I needed to be by her side. What if she needed me, and I was not there? Shortly after I arrived, we had a visit from the doctor, who said that they would move her out of ICU in a little while to a private room. I sat and had a long visit with her, until she slipped back into much-needed sleep. I sat in the waiting room surrounded by family listening to talk of answered prayers, relief, and much concern. The tears were hard to hold back; I guess the great sense of relief, the tension, the fear, all of it together, everything that I had experienced and had never felt before, they all came rushing back. It had been a long few days.

She was moved to a private room and began the long road to recovery. Family and friends made their way through, as she tried to rest. At one point, she fell asleep, and I moved my chair into the hallway, closed the door, and headed off family members, friends and neighbors, well-wishers who all had wonderful intentions. My goal was to let her rest and keep her room quiet. My sweet wife needed to rest, to recover, and make her way back to me. I did not care if I upset someone, and I could tell I did. Uncles and aunts who had come to see Barbie sat and talked to me, waiting on me to say, "OK, come on in," but I did not say that. No one mattered but Barbie, and I was determined to see to it that whatever she needed she got, and now she needed rest.

The doctor came in first thing the next morning and informed us that she could go home that afternoon. My mother expressed her displeasure at the fact that they were sending her home a little more than thirty hours after surgery; after all, we lived out in the county 35 minutes from the closest hospital. The doctor commented, "Why, it's just brain surgery?" That answer did little to appease my mother, who was visibly upset; she knew that I would be left alone to care for her, and she thought I wasn't ready. I often wonder how much the fact that we had no insurance played into the decision, but nevertheless, for the first time in my life, I was about to become a caregiver, and I was determined to be the best possible choice for the job.

We made our way home that evening, a stop by the pharmacy to fill prescriptions and get medical supplies, Barbie was doing well but seemed to be in a fog; I thought – thought, hoped, prayed – that as she recovered that would pass. We were immediately set upon by many well-wishing neighbors bringing food over for us, in the country when someone dies, is sick, real sad or anything else that someone, especially the women of the community feels they may be able to help, they cook and bring it to you. It is a wonderful thing to live in a place where people know you, care for you, and want to help you. We had casseroles, hams, pies and cakes, but what we really had was the knowledge that we had friends and family who cared for us and cared enough to want to show it. The men also would come by or send word by their wife, "If you need anything all you have to do is call." I knew they meant it; a call or two and I would have tractors rolling over the farm taking care of our needs.

We lived in a small community; there were farms broken by three small villages established years ago when twenty miles was a long way to travel. All the needs were addressed in these villages, but today they are just a few houses, small general stores, maybe a gas pump. Everyone knows each other, and we are all tied together either by commerce, church, school or relation. Most of the people I started first grade with still live within five or six miles. It is a wonderful thing to live in a place like that; it is sad to see that it seems to be going by the wayside. Still, even places like this are not as close as they were fifteen or twenty years ago. We should all make it a point, myself included, to go out and meet our neighbors. We will be richer for it.

Chapter 4
Our Community

I place much emphasis on the importance of community family and friends, and the community we live in is typical of many small farming communities around our country. We live along Symmes Creek in southern Ohio. There are small communities every three to seven miles; these are spread out among small family farms that range from 25 to a thousand acres, with most being around one 150 to 250 acres. These particular small communities were founded in the mid 1800s; at that time travel was difficult, with the only roads being stage coach routes, which were little more than wagon tracks wore into the soil, so each community developed a self-sufficiency that has endured, but is beginning to be lost in this era of easy travel. I read history accounts of difficult travel between the villages of Arabia and Waterloo due to the only road being in a state of disrepair, and that was a distance of only three miles. As I looked into the history of the area, I found that both of these communities at one time had doctors, drug stores, blacksmiths, taverns, general merchandise stores, saddle makers, flour mills (both steam- and water-driven), and even hotels; they were totally self-sufficient with the local families having only each other to depend on. in those days travel even between these two close communities was difficult, partly because each was on a different side of the creek.

Our farm lies close to Arabia, and I attended grade school at Waterloo; Barbie attended one of the other small grade schools that were spread throughout the area. We both attended the same high school, but I had graduated by the time she got there. The village of Waterloo and its school have a very interesting history; at one time in addition to the business listed above there was a movie 25 five to a hundred, there are few businesses to speak of anymore, only scattered small local stores, many doubling as a restaurant and a gas station, but those are fading away. Today the trip has become easy to Ironton, Ashland or Gallipolis where major retailers can be found and prices that make the trip seem worthwhile, but the cost of local business being lost also seems high. Even though commerce is disappearing at an alarming rate, the community spirit still exists, and the habit of relying and depending on each other is still alive and well. Although it is no longer always on display, it still comes out when one is in need.

At one time, all of the little villages had Grange halls, churches, taverns, or the school house, where everyone met from time to time. These were the heart of the community and served to strengthen those ties. Today the Grange halls sit abandoned, the taverns are gone with only a small store and a few tables remaining, many of the churches have been abandoned and are used for hay storage with the ones still open serving only a small portion of the population. I fear that the future generation may never know the close community spirit that abounds all across our great nation, the same that has been instrumental in helping us through our times of trouble. Today, we often see large fundraising drives that are very helpful as the savings dwindle and the bills loom like a dark cloud , but those cannot compare to someone who visits, gives you a hug, and cries with you if needed.

Our family moved there the year that I was born. In an area with generations of families that have always lived together and depended on each other, or in some cases disliked, each other for generations, we were slow to be accepted into the community. It seemed that everyone was related by blood or marriage or tied together by the long years of families existing side by side, but eventually we were accepted as part of this wonderful community. The older generation had all been born on the small family farms that dotted the area in a time when those small farms provided a living and sustained the family; many were the farms that contained less than fifty acres that provided the means to raise a family. The older generation had all went to school and grown up together, and for the most part were still around. Our Janitor at Waterloo when I was in grade school had been part of the local basketball team that a quarter of a century earlier had earned some degree of fame; they were known as the Waterloo Wonders and won multiple state championships in the 1940s. They played college and pro teams and came out victorious more often than not. They were known to have three players on the court with the other two playing marbles on the side lines or ate hot dogs in the stands while the game went on. They had become widely known not only for their antics but their ability to win games. Our janitor with a couple of warm-up shots could still make many consecutive baskets shooting from the opposite foul line through the rafters and into the basket. He would entertain young ones who cared to listen with stories of learning to play with a ball made of rolled up gloves and a coffee tin for a basket; one of the things that had made the team so good was its ability to move the ball by passing, a skill learned out of necessity, since their ball did not bounce. He and his wife also ran the local store that joined our farm as I grew up, and the lady who lived across the street, from the store, had been one of two cheerleaders for the same basketball team; this wonderful lady was also my third grade teacher and Sunday school teacher at our local church. The remainder of that team still lived either in those two villages or on farms surrounding them. Their families were for the most part working on the farms and at public jobs; many were the teachers, bus drivers and coaches who were molding the next generation in the community, in which they had lived their whole lives.

Growing up, I think of how different it was from today. On the school bus the driver had the right and moreover was expected to require the children to respect them and their fellow passengers; there would usually be a wooden paddle hanging beside them to enforce this rule if needed, and it would be used without hesitation. Fights and bullying did not happen on the bus, as they were stopped before they could start, usually by the driver who had grown up with the parents of the kids on the bus. The same was to be expected at school. Respect was the rule of the day, and if discipline was required at school, word would usually reached home before the student did, and another dose of discipline would be waiting there also. There were o complaints because you disciplined my child but apologies that they had to.

I always smile when recalling the day that we were on the bus and my neighbors, two brothers, started fighting. We were out on a dirt road, close to nothing, and the bus driver, who also happened to be the uncle of the two brothers, stopped the bus. He asked the older brother to step outside, saying "I need to talk to you." As the brother stepped off of the bus, the door closed and the bus drove off, the younger brother waving out the back window as his big brother disappeared into the cloud of dust. It was not the bus driver who was in trouble when the student eventually finished his long walk home. If a fight broke out at school, the response was usually, "You boys go out in the grass so someone does not get hurt." It was understood that certain things had to be figured out for everyone to get along and become that tight community we lived in. We were shaped by a very different generation and culture, and time was reshaping all of them.

By this time the family farm was fading from the countryside, Oh they are still here, but now those operating them were steel workers, postal employees, foundry workers, pipe liners, construction workers or employed by local business owners. The twenty mile drive to town is overlooked and to survive outside income is required. The farm still supplied much of the family's needs, but money was also required, something that was not as needed in as great of an amount as times past. As I grew up, there were no longer farms operating without some outside income, gone were the days of bartering with the neighbors or local businessmen for what they could not produce. But even though the economy was changing, the strong sense of community was not; everyone had grown up together, and many of their parents had also; they were all there for each other, the local gatherings were a thing of the past, but with added work off of the farm there was less time to socialize and less need for places to do so.

When I was small, the common practice would be for dad and two neighbors to work together on harvest. They would move from farm to farm each bringing their equipment and working until the job was completed; there was still the camaraderie, but it was shared in the field. There were visits at the local stores or the feed store where a chance meeting would result in shared stories and talk of how crops were looking, of crop and livestock prices, and the news of the community, many times over a cold bottle of pop from the machine, and when the drink was finished, there was work to be done. These meeting would replace the larger get-togethers that once were commonplace in the area. I read of the old community gatherings, over occasions like the Fourth of July, where hundreds of families would all come together to celebrate. Now it is a drive to town to gather among a group of strangers to watch a large firework display, eat something bought from someone in a booth or a van, and drive home, interacting only with the people who came with you. In those days, it was a large community event with a pot luck dinner or picnic; the object was not to watch some elaborate display but to socialize with friends and neighbors, to forge those bonds that are quickly being lost in today's society.

Today as the next generation matures and moves off to chase dreams, many of whom settle in large cities and towns among others doing the same, and most do not even know their closest neighbors. We are missing out on something that has been taken for granted by our past generations. And it is not only in those large cities and towns; I am sad to say it is occurring in the small country communities as well. Most of the people I went to school with still live in our community, but we have let the cares of life separate us, and most do not visit or talk. We no longer run into each other at the local feed or hardware stores because it is easy to get to the large ones in town. We are still bound by that sense of community, but I fear that we may be the last generation in this area to have that joy. It is of our own doing; I am ashamed to say that I do not know some of the folks who now live in the area, people have moved in, and I have not taken the time to visit and welcome them here. It seems that making a living, dealing with our and my families, business, and problems is my focus. I lament the loss of community but realize that I am contributing to it. There is still very much the sense of duty to help our fellow man when times of catastrophic loss occur, and this is a great thing, but it is not as personal as it could or should be.

I think of the old Farm Field Days that the local farmers would take turns hosting. There would be beans and cornbread cooked in large cast iron pots for dinner, pies and cakes baked by the local ladies, and various refreshments. For all the farm families and any of the community that wanted, crop production would be displayed and viewed while ideas were exchanged, but a lot of sitting on hay bales and just visiting took place. It was a rare day off that we all gathered together and enjoyed each other's company. I recall one day shortly after we leased the farm that our family hosted one of these field days. Several of us men were gathered talking around the bean pots that were cooking. The old gentleman who was cooking the bean was a veteran of many field days, often cooking the beans. As we talked, a large roach ran out of the pipe frame and made its way across the horizontal pipe holding the large pots. We all watched and silently rooted for it to make it. It passed over the pot of brown beans, and as it got about half way over the pot of white beans (my favorite), the heat got to it, and it plunged into the pot. With a casualness that relayed that this was not the first time, the old man dipped it out and tossed it into the fire. We all swallowed a little hard thinking about past bowls of beans this chef had prepared for us, and I had the brown beans that day. These days also have faded into the past, to be replaced with online forums, message boards and the so-called social networks. I am saddened by the future that is unfolding for our youth, many of who count friends by likes or friend-me notices. They may never know the kind of friendship that will lead someone to get out of bed and come along beside you in the middle of the night in your time of need. Many of these networks will pull together and help financially, and that is a great thing, but it is no substitute for those who will stand with you, cry with you, and laugh with you, and just give you a hug to let you know they care.

We have been truly blessed to grow up in the time and the area that we have, when people have come together in the good times and in the bad, who care for each other and are quick to show it, I still talk to my mother and hear, "I am going to run their dinner up to them." We had a wonderful lady and friend bring us up a homecooked meal just the other day. It was very good, but it was not the food that we were filled with; it was the outpouring of love from a neighbor the we savored. And it is this community that comes along side of Barbie and I in our time of greatest need, the phone calls to us and our parents to continually monitor her progress, the meals that were brought in, the field work that was done on my behalf, the donations made at Barbie's benefit, the numerous donations from local churches, many that I did not know, but someone who one of us had grown up with attended. I do not go anywhere in the area without hearing "How is Barbie doing?" I tell them of the details, good or bad, because they have ask out of love and because they care.

We always try to help in any way we can, if it be donating

something for raffle or just making donations, but we try when health permits to show up, because we learned, being there means as much as anything, showing others that you are willing to take time out of your life to be in theirs when they need that is what touched me and Barbie in our time of need. Money will come and go, bills will do the same, but the love shown to other in their time of need will endure. Yes, we are truly blessed to live in the small community of Arabia/Waterloo/Wilgus, and we are forever grateful for being a part of the lives of each and every one, and to have each as a part of our lives. We are much richer because of the friendship and love that is shown in each smile, each inquiry to someone's health, and each pie or cake, baked with love and sent for comfort.

Chapter 5
Recovery, the Darkness Deepens, and the Light Shines

After we arrived at home and both began to get some much needed rest, I called my boss and informed him of what we were facing, and gave back any work that I had to do so I could stay home and take care of Barbie. I could not leave her alone, and hiring someone to come in and take care of her while I worked was not an option, so the only choice was for me to do it. As the days began to pass, my concern deepened; she was doing physically fine, but the fog was not lifting. She could not grasp the words she needed when talking, and the names of longtime friends and neighbors would not come to her. She would tell me to "Look at the thermometer and see what time it was" or to "get some ice out of the stove." The words were there but all mixed up. Sometimes as she would try to talk to me she would get stuck, and a look of frustration often was on her face. She did continue to recover well from her surgery. Her food of choice was watermelon, and fortunately my parents had a large patch that was just ripening, daily visits from my mom and dad to bring her melon were a comfort. Her grandfather also began making almost daily visits, a long-time Baptist preacher who had lost his wife several years before began to be a much relied upon source of comfort for me, he would stop by to visit and spend time with me alone in a field or somewhere; I would talk, and he would listen. This is something we all tend to forget from time to time, often people just need someone to listen, or just sit silently with them. I spent days working and trying to make her comfortable and aid in her recovery, taking care of our son, and thinking about what was to come, and how we would face it, it was wonderful to be there for her; I am thankful that I was able to help her when she needed me. I spent a lot of time talking to her, watching television with her and doing everything that I could to give our life and her condition any semblance of normal, even though it was far from it.

As the days passed, she began to get out and to attempt to resume her normal life. One day we were out taking a short walk. We were down at the end of the driveway by a barn when she walked over and picked up a brick and carried it to a mud hole in the driveway, stood at the edge of the puddle and pitched the brick in. She was instantly covered with patches of mud from head to toe. At first I had to laugh until I noticed her look of total disbelief and confusion. She had no idea that the result of throwing that brick into the mud would be mud splashing. I felt very sad for her and went over to help her, and to try to explain what had happened. We went to the house and got cleaned up. I realized I was going to have to watch and help her very closely, for many of the things we learned growing up and take for granted, she had lost. She was going to need to learn a great deal all over, and with her short-term memory compromised, she had her work cut out for her.

As we went through the days, she steadily improved. Her health and appetite continued to improve, and she was nearing her old self physically, as family and friends came by to visit it was painful to watch her struggle to hold a conversation, she could communicate, and the thoughts were clear, but there seemed to be a road block when looking for some words. She quickly began to fall into a habit of looking to me when she would hang up on a word; everyone was gracious and held conversations with her as normal, and the lovely smile that had been a constant part of who she was would return now and then; it was good to see. That was a much needed ray of light into a time when all else seemed to be very dark. It was clear that she was not going to be the same; the only question was how bad was it going to be. I tried to put these thought out of my mind and focus on taking care of her, trying to do what I could to see that she healed as quick and as well as possible.

At the urging of my parents and their local pastor, we decided to go to church with them; after all, I had been praying, and it appeared that prayers were answered – she had survived surgery and was recovering. This was probably a week-and-a-half after her surgery. She had begun to walk daily and was desperately trying to get back to normal, to regain her life, and we even had decided to go to the local high school football game that Friday to watch our boy play in the band. Church on the following Wednesday went well; we were received with love and surrounded by people who genuinely cared. This was great, neighbors and family had been wonderful, but people who we considered friends were noticeably absent in our lives. It seems when really bad health events happen that true friends are discovered and those who were not are lost. This came as quite a shock to us, we thought that we had a lot of friends, but it was quite obvious what is meant by fair weather friends. The football game also went very well, the struggle with conversation was more apparent, as there were many who wanted to talk and see how she was doing, "what was their name" was a question I answered many times as well-wishers walked off, people she had went to school with and known all of her life were known to her but the names were lost, but our thought was if this is the worst thing, we will be OK. We were confident that if she regained her physical health, then we could work together and she could get closer to normal, hopeful that the old Barbie was still in there and we could coax her back.

The two weeks between her surgery and the follow-up appointment finally passed, so we went to the doctor to hear the pathology report and get her stitches removed. This appointment fell on my thirty-eighth birthday, a day we will never forget. We waited in the backroom of the doctor's office, nervous but encouraged by her quick physical recovery; her health was great, she was strong and doing great. The doctor came in and greeted us, he ask how she was doing and walked around behind here and begin to remove stitches, comments on how well she was healing up brightened our visit, then it came. He told us that the tumor she had was an oligodendroglioma and that some the cells were anaplastic We did not know what this all meant, but his demeanor spoke volumes. He asked her, "Have you ever had a vacation?" She said no, and he told her that she should take one because this would be what took her life. He explained as the tears began to roll down our faces that anaplasticeant malignant and that it made this a grade-three tumor; it also meant that he needed to go back in – and soon – and resect more of the tumor to try to get to clear borders. The surgery was set for two weeks from that date. As the visit wrapped up, we were stunned. We walked by the front desk without stopping and out to the car. We were devastated, and just held each other and cried and cried, for what seemed to be a long time.

When we gained enough composure, we began the long drive home. Barbie wanted to go out for my birthday dinner, saying that she did not want to ruin my day. This was typical of her personality; she always thought more of others than her needs. I told her I did not feel like going out, and she agreed. My head swam as I drove, nearing the point of passing out. Deep breaths and concentration kept me conscious as I drove. She just sat and sobbed. When we got home we broke down again, held each other and cried until there were no more tears. I had to go down and break the devastating news to my parents. I walked the mile to their house, trying to catch my breath, trying to stop my head from spinning; this was not what we expected, she was recovering so well. Barbie and I each needed a little time to process things. I cried as I walked, and she cried at the house. I told my parents, and they cried. I don't know how I looked as I walked home but one of our neighbors who I had known all of her life passed by, as I walked up our road, and just by looking at me from behind she went home and told her mother something was wrong. Calls came in to my parents, and the news quickly spread.

The next day broke, and Barbie got up and said, "Let's take a walk, I need to get in shape for this next surgery, I am going to beat this thing." This would prove to be her battle plan. She would demonstrate her commitment to it over and over again, one day to be sad, then the fight was on. I was taken aback; I knew that she was courageous, and that she would not give up, but I was surprised that so soon after a terminal prognosis, she had put the news behind her and was ready to fight for her life. So we began walking each day, and she started training for her upcoming fight. I heard very few words about dying or this taking her life, that was not an option, she would win, we would walk together, and I would walk alone later. I walked many miles with tear-filled eyes, worrying about my bride.

My prayer life picked up again. I had been thankful for the outcome of her first surgery, but now the prospect of another one scared me, after all, if she came out worse, would she even be able to communicate, think, function. I prayed that the Lord would save her while she had the mental faculties to accept Him. Sunday morning came, and we went to church. We were surrounded by the loving congregation; they cried with us and prayed for us. The preacher, a longtime friend and a genuine man of God, was in the pulpit. He preached his message out of:

Now we know that God heareth not sinners: but if any man be a worshipper of God, and doeth his will, him he heareth. (Joh 9:31)

He brought out the point that you could be in the middle of a storm and you may need the Lord to listen more than you ever have in your life, but if you were out of fellowship and in a sinful state, then the Bible says He was not hearing. I knew that the preacher was talking to me, that God was talking to me, I was sorry for the way I had lived the last twenty years, separated from God and sinning against him. I needed Him in my life, not only because I knew He was the only one who could heal Barbie, save her soul, but I needed Him because I could not face this on my own. I was at a

crossroads in my life, I would either fall on my knees and follow God, or fall on my face and rely on the things I had been
involved in for the past twenty years. I shuddered to think
how my life would have been had I went that way. As the
altar call was given, I stepped out and went forward to re-
dedicate my life to Him. I instantly felt better; I knew when I
prayed He was listening and we had a lot to talk about,
twenty years of regrets and a desperate need. After I got
home that evening, I began clearing out some of the old
habits I had fell into, as the days past I thought about slipping
back into some of them, as I had in times past;the message
was impressed on me very clearly that if I wanted His help, I
needed to be serious about this, I needed to make the Lord of
my life and put down the things that had kept me away so
long, or He would take her. Now I do not believe the Lord
makes a habit of speaking audibly, and I do not think that He
did to me, but it was just as plain as if He did, and at that
instant I laid down those things and by His grace have not
looked back.

We continued with her training, routine walking, and trying to get back to where she had been before her first
surgery. We attended Church on Wednesday, and I was
blessed to be there. Later that week, we got an appointment
with a doctor at Ohio University Hospital in Columbus, this
was about a two-hour drive from our house. He was by
reputation one of the authorities on the type of tumor that
Barbie had. Our visit was very depressing. Our local surgeon
was a godly man who told us that he would not put a time on
her prognosis, that it was in the hands of God, and he would
not venture to go there. But this doctor had no such
reservations; he informed us that she would have six months,
maybe a year, to live at the most. While the radiologist had

told us that he felt he could help her live five years, this doctor said flatly, "That will not happen." We had another tearful drive home, but Barbie did not accept this timeline, saying, "I am going to beat this thing and live."

The Sunday after we got home, we went to Sunday School then Church that night. As the altar call was given, Barbie looked up at her grandpa, who was on the other side of her, then she looked at me, with a very stern look on her face, leaving me quite puzzled. When we got home and her grandpa had left, I asked her about the look. She said, "Did grandpa say go on?" Now, her grandpa was very hard of hearing, usually with his hearing aids turned up to the point the you could hear them whistle, and whispering was not part of his vocabulary, so I could very confidently answer, "No, he did not." Then she said, "Did you?" I said no, and she looked on thoughtfully. I told her that if she was hearing "go on" during the altar call, that maybe that is what she should do.

As we went through the week, her resolve grew. She walked daily and gained strength at an amazing pace; she was training for the fight of her life. I had been out working on the farm and came home one day and found her sitting on the porch step with her head down. I asked what she was doing. She said, "I am telling the Lord all the things that I have done." My heart leapt, and I told her to go on as I walked in the house. As the week rolled on, Wednesday finally came and the evening Church service. At the altar call, she again looked at Grandpa, then me, then she stepped out and went to the altar and accepted Jesus as her savior. Thank you Lord! As stated earlier, I do not hear the Lord speak audibly, but Barbie contends to this day and will until her last, that the Lord spoke to her on more than one occasion that way. It occurred to me that he knew his children and spoke to each in the way that can personally be understood, and maybe that with what she was going through that was what He needed to do.

As our hearts leapt for joy, we still faced the stark realization that another brain surgery loomed closer every day. Barbie kept up her training and readied herself for the fight of her life. This weighed on me – the medical bills that were piling up weighed on me, the household bills and all of the rest of life was still there, but now there was a bright light that shined through the darkness. We had both officially repented; now that just meant to turn from one direction and start going another, which is exactly what we had done. We had stopped following the desires of our minds and bodies, to the best of our abilities, and started doing our best to follow the Lord. It is a wonderful feeling to know that your prayers are heard, and in times when you feel there is no one that you can talk to, that there is no one who understands, you can take it to Him.

Therefore if any man be in Christ, he is a new creature: old things are passed away; behold, all things are become new. (2Co 5:17)

For he hath made him to be sin for us, who knew no sin; that we might be made the righteousness of God in him. (2Co 5:21)

We both felt good to be new creatures, our old running around "friends" had forsaken us, and now we had a new one who promised to never leave, and along came a group of people who not only said that they loved us but showed us so. Our lives had turned around, and it felt good, but all of our problems had not gone away. We still had every one of them, but now they seemed different.

Chapter 6
Surgery No. 2

As the surgery approached at what seemed to be a dizzying pace, we continued to ready ourselves as much as possible. I reflected on the fact that while in the waiting room during surgery each minute seems to last and hour and during the month between surgery number one and two that each day seemed to take only an hour.Only one short month had passed since our lives had changed forever; at that point, it still seemed that our lives were turned upside down and all had changed for the worse, it occurs to me that when in times like these it is extremely hard to see the good that is mixed in with the bad, I believe it is always there, but until we grow and learn through this life we can only see it by looking back from the other side of the storm.

And we know that all things work together for good to them that love God, to them who are the called according to his purpose. (Ro 8:28)

This verse quickly became one of my favorite passages; it speaks to the fact that we do not know the future, so at the present time, we cannot always tell what is a good thing and what is not, this is a lesson that I would learn as the years rolled by.

The alarm clock sounded, and the day had arrived. I again struggled to put on a brave front, and I am sure, although you could not tell it that Barbie was doing the same. Our son, showing he was his mother's son, had the same brave face on that we did, no tears, no worry showing. We sure were good actors. We got ready, and after the long drive walked into the hospital at 6 a.m. I witnessed another astounding feat of bravery, as my lovely wife squared her shoulders and without so much as a tear walked into the hospital and back into pre-op to begin her preparation for surgery. Again many of our family members were present, and more would drift in as the first hour passed. Our pastor was there and his family; we again tried to pass the time by distraction, while we waited time seemed to pass when we should have been taken back to see here prior to surgery. I asked the nurse what was taking so long and was informed that she had already been taken back, and that she had ask that no one come back. Later Barbie told me she did not want everyone to see her after they prepped her because we would just worry more; this was typical of Barbie – even in her worse times, her concern is not centered on herself.

We talked in disbelief about what had just happened and tried to not think about the fact that we could have missed our last opportunity to see and talk to her. Again the clocks around the world began to malfunction as minutes took hours to pass. There was still the same anxiety filling my heart, but the loneliness was not as profound; I still spent the time in the restroom on my knees, but my prayer had changed somewhat. Oh, I still pleaded for a good outcome, and for my wonderful wife to make a full return to me. But I no longer had the feeling of despair that came from knowing that I could have seen her for the last time or wondered if anyone was listening to my prayers. There was also a big difference in the fact that this surgery had not taken me by surprise like the last one had. We knew we were coming this time and were as prepared as we could be. Sitting in the waiting room, my mind began to drift again. I looked at our son and thought of how proud Barbie was of him, of the little league games when in the stands she shouted encouragement which seemed to annoy and embarrass him, but she could not hold it back. I thought about the basketball games, the band, whatever he did, it did not matter if he was good or bad at it, she was his number one fan. I smiled a little as I thought of when we watched his first attempt at extreme sports. He was five or so, and was out riding his bike, I happened to look out the bathroom window in time to see him with a ramp set up to jump the three foot wide creek that bordered out yard. Barbie was walking by, and I said, "Come here, we might as well watch because it's too late to stop him." As he was just starting his approach, his front wheel left the ramp and immediately started to drop. As the back wheel left the ramp, the front hit the ditch, and he was sent on a short flight over the handle bars. He got up, looked around and stood awhile, then dragged his ramp back into the barn and for at least a while, ended his daredevil career. As the hours continued to crawl by, loved ones tried to comfort each other, and again what was scheduled for a six-hour surgery turned into eight, and everyone was getting worn out from the long hours of stress. There were many comings and goings throughout the day, and sometime during this long day, I had a visit from a lady in the financial office of the hospital who asks me to visit her after everything settled down.

Finally, the doctor made his way out and ask to speak with

me. Again my heart raced. Was this normal, was something wrong? He explained that all had went well; he again had awoken her on the table, and she responded well. He told me of the golden rule of "good in, good out" and how much better she had started this surgery then the last. Family and friends listened intently as I relayed the report. Many filed by and gave hugs and extended offers to do anything that was needed or in their power, I appreciated it more than could be expressed. As I waited with the closest of family for her to get out of recovery, so I could see her, I again was relieved and thankful that she had once again survived and hopeful that maybe we would have more time together, but still the grim prognosis and the uncertainty of what our future would hold – would she ever be able to function on her own? – filled my thoughts and loomed over our lives like a black cloud.

The recovery went much the same as last time, the terrible day in ICU hooked to all manner of monitor and machine, the coming out from under Anastasia and recognizing everyone, the long night of restless sleep in the ICU waiting room. But again, she did amazingly well and way before my mother thought she should, we were on the way home. The fog lingered for a couple of days, but her recovery was a little more complete. As she progressed, communication became easier, names came a little better but not all the way, she was left with little short-term memory and few inhibitions but had the ability to function and do more of her day-to-day activities. She was very weak and tired easily, and I still felt it necessary to be there to help her. I was falling into the role of caregiver. I was lucky that I had always been able to cook, cleaning was a little tougher on me, but I was raised with the saying, "A man's gotta do what a man's gotta do," and I did.

The follow-up doctor appointment came and went with no surprises this time. Recovery was on track or a little ahead, she was healing very well, and the next step of her treatment was scheduled – a full course of radiation treatments where she would receive the maximum allowable radiation to the area of her tumor. We went in, and she had a mask made to hold her still while taking the treatments. The treatments stretched out over months in which five days a week, we would travel in the morning and then get a treatment that lasted only a few minutes. I spent a lot of time getting comfort from the Scriptures while waiting. Christmas came and went, and time rolled by, but all in all she tolerated radiation very well, with only fatigue to deal with, she would daily fall asleep at 2 p.m. for about an hour regardless of what was going on for the day. She was adamant that life re-turn to normal as much as possible, so we attended local football games that fall, where our son played in the band, and tried to do all the things that people in our position typically do. We spent many evening with me reading the Bible to her only to look up and see she was deep in sleep. She finished her treatments and had regained a lot of her function and abilities, but sadly apparent was the fact that there would be a permanent change. We were determined to live the life we had and to be thankful for all. We visited the oncologist next, and it was suggested that she start on a chemo regiment. It was about this time that the fact we had no insurance begin to weigh heavily on Barbie and she would routinely ask, "How much will this cost?" I would tell her it did not matter, determined to do whatever was needed to get her the treatment to keep her alive and with me. The oncologist, a wonderful man, told her that he made enough treating patients that he could afford to treat one for free every now and then and that he would just let his drug reps know that he needed some samples, and there would be no charge. Barbie at that time had beautiful long hair that she dearly loved; we were told that hair loss could be a side effect, and if she cut her hair it would not be as bad. She asked me if I would cut it for her, and I did. She stood in the bathroom and cried while I cut twelve to fifteen inches from her hair. She took two doses and was deathly sick both times, spending most of the night on her knees in the bathroom. She called me into the bedroom and told me that "If I only have six months to live, I am not going to spend it all throwing up," and the decision was made to end the treatment. I was saddened by her decision but could understand; I was also very relieved that she was now able to make that decision on her own.

Now the road to recovery was to begin. The second surgery and the extensive course of radiation had left her very fatigued, but she did bounce back after surgery and started walking again, but not as soon as the first time; it seems that one of the lingering effects of the radiation and maybe the tumor would be fatigue that was to stay with her. The days of her getting out on the farm and working in the fields were coming to an end. Before she got sick, Barbie would work in the fields beside me as long as we needed to, when we would need to hire people to work. Many times we would all work side by side and seldom would anyone be able to complete the job ahead of her. This was always a joy to her; she worked the farm, kept the house, paid the bills, and did anything that was needed for us to make it. She would continue to be an amazing wife and do many of these things, but as I learned later from reading journals, it was much harder and left her very tired. One of her enduring

qualities was that she never complained, and must be pressed to find out when something was bothering her, so at the
time I missed much of this in the process of doing what had
to be done.

I was beginning to hit my stride as a stay-at-home dad – I
was cooking, cleaning, running the errands, and trying to be
there for her every need. As she recovered, she would insist
on reclaiming much of her role. She was also well enough
that I could leave her home alone for a while, so I resumed
working on the farm and doing some things outside. It felt
good, was a step back to our life. Church was a regular part of
our life now and we had a new pastor; he and his family
would soon become some of our most dear and trusted
friends. He often told us with tear-filled eyes of the day he
met Barbie. He came the day after her second surgery, and
upon greeting her he casually asked, "How are you doing
Barbie?" to which she answered, "I am dying." This was one
of the few days I ever remember he saying that; it was on one
of her rare, out of the fight days. His wife and Barbie were the
same age and shared the same birthday, so a yearly birthday
dinner tradition began.

The shadow of her prognosis was hard to shake, I found
myself searching the Internet for survivor stories, looking for
some hope, for someone to say, "I beat it," there were a few,
but finding any that stretched past five years was difficult.
But that did not matter, I believed Barbie when she said that
she was going to beat it, and I also knew and believed what I
read:

*Ah Lord GOD! behold, thou hast made the heaven and the
earth by thy great power and stretched out arm, and there is
nothing too hard for thee... (Jer 32:17)*

We are also told that with God all things are possible, and I knew that if he wished that he could heal her with no effort. I just did not know if it was His will or if it was the best thing in our lives. One of the hardest things for me to learn was to pray that His will would be done, and for years I prayed that He would do my will, and that was to heal my beloved.

Even though the light had begun to shine into our lives, this was still a very dark time. We had faith and believed what we read, but that did not change the fact that our lives were in total disarray. For example, our son was beginning to have problems in school. He routinely tested in the top few percent of the country, but we had to press to keep him from having failing grades. I know that even though he did not let on, the situation at home was weighing heavily on him, and his life was spiraling out of control just like ours was. After all, he was facing the loss of the one constant in his young life – his mother. This phase in his life would last several years, until after he had graduated high school. He would become more distant for several years, finally as we tend to do, with maturity the realization that everyone was doing their best in a hard situation would sink in and a new phase of a wonderful relationship would begin. I think of a time when Barbie was strangely prophetic. One day, long before this all began, we talked about the future, and she made a strange comment for a young healthy person: "As long as I can see my son graduate, I will be happy." This took me a little off guard, and as I look back, even more so.

Chapter 7
Looking Back Through the Darkness to See the Light

As I mentioned earlier, sometimes you have to get past a certain point in your life before you can look back and see good things and the blessings in your life. This is also when it is often easier to see the Lord working in your life.

Just after the second surgery, I was at our local county store and the lady who runs the store, also a longtime family friend, was asking me about Barbie, then she looked at me and said, "Don't worry about your tobacco crop in the field." I was a little puzzled because I had not; it was the furthest thing from my mind, even though it was a big part of my yearly income. I just did not have the time or desire to worry about it; I had more important things on my mind. She then told me, "I am going to take care of it." She then told me that she had arranged a crew to come over and house my crop for me, totally at her expense. During the next week, there were many neighbors and friends on the farm; I do not think many of them required any payment, and I will forever be in their debt. My crop was housed, and I was able to put on a cookout for all who helped and Barbie was able to attend and we all had a good time. We talked about many things and always they expressed how sorry they were, and the desire to help in any way possible, I choked back tears most of that day; The talks with concerned friends and neighbors proved to be harder then I thought they would be, to this day nothing hits home like and affects me like someone who sincerely cares and offers their help, I realize how lucky I am to have those people in my life.

During this time, I also met with the lady from the financial office of the hospital. We reviewed my assets and my income, and I relayed how we had been working to build us a house and that we had lost two consecutive crops, and how that had seemed like a dark time in our lives. I think often how in those days it seemed like the worst thing that could happen, but I still did not have a proper definition of the word *problem*. Because of those two years, we were living in a rental house that belonged to my dad; we did not have any assets to speak of, so a zero went into that column. Then since I had taken a contract job, and upon Barbie getting sick could not afford to hire an caregiver, I was forced to stop working. I was then unemployed and a zero also went into that column. So what had seemed as the darkest time in our lives at one time was the Lord preparing the way for a truly dark time to come.

Fear thou not; for I am with thee: be not dismayed; for I am thy God: I will strengthen thee; yea, I will help thee; yea, I will uphold thee with the right hand of my righteousness. (ISA 41:10)

Since we had no assets and I had no job, she filled out the

paperwork for assistance, and we qualified. This became retroactive to the first emergency room visit and what I estimated to be close to a half million dollars in medical bills were wiped away. Now to some this may not seem to be an unusual occurrence, but we have always worked for anything that we have gotten. Dad worked a full-time job and saved for his dream, to own a farm; growing up, there were times when all we had to eat was grown on the farm, I smile when I think, what most people see as something you eat when you can't afford anything else, bologna, was something I saw as a treat. We raised cattle and hogs, there were usually a few chickens around, so all that was available, but you had to buy bologna. So when the bills started piling up, I saw my future in front of me, all dreams were replaced with paying medical bills off, the future on this front had looked bleak, and I did not spend much time thinking about it. I had to do whatever Barbie needed, but the thought did haunt me. I could lose her and still have a lifetime of bills to pay on, but that was not an issue. I would do all that I could to get he the help she needed, in this I see the hand of God working in my life long before Barbie got sick.

The righteous cry, and the LORD heareth, and delivereth them out of all their troubles. The LORD is nigh unto them that are of a broken heart; and saveth such as be of a contrite spirit. Many are the afflictions of the righteous: but the LORD delivereth him out of them all. (Ps 34:17-19)

I fit into the group of "righteous" not because of what I had done, or how good I was; the fact is I was just the opposite, but I had accepted Jesus as my savior when I was twelve and it is his righteousness that is looked upon.

I still was not able to work, but there was a great cloud lifted from over our head, then shortly after, the daughter of the Lady who "took care of my tobacco crop" asked if she could have a benefit to raise money to help Barbie. I had known this girl since she was a baby, and even though we do not share blood, we are family. We agreed and thanked her from the bottom of our heart. The whole neighborhood turned out in support, and much was raised. Local churches also gave us love offerings, and even in the time of our greatest distress, the Lord taught us that he could provide and sustain us through this. The Benefit was a great time; we had singing, games and a pig roast, it was the first time that Barbie had been able to really do anything to enjoy herself since this had all begun, and was a much-needed distraction. There were games, raffles and an auction, where people brought things, anything, and it was auctioned off, the meal was free with donations accepted, and again the outpouring of love choked me up. At one time when the rain was falling gently, a man was singing "Blue Eyes Crying in the Rain" it got to me a little, and my blue eyes were. At that time my Dad said something that was profound and has come to pass many times over: "Dave, there are people here feeling sorry for Barbie and thinking that she is going to die, and have no idea that their time will come before hers." He went on to explain how we are all in the Lord's hands and will go when He calls; we all have an appointment set, and we will not be late.

And as it is appointed unto men once to die, but after this the judgment... (Heb 9:27)

Two weeks did not pass before a young lady who we knew

and that who was there lost her life in a motorcycle accident – and since then it would be hard to number those who have gone out of this life who were there. So through this time in our life, the Lord using family, friends and community provided for all of our needs. The cloud was not lifted, but the light shone through, and it was comprehended.

As time moved on, we started to regain some since of normalcy. Barbie continued to improve, her strength began to return, her ability to converse improved, and she was able to go about her day. Just before the cold weather set in, we were able to get the vacation that doctor suggested. We and two of her cousins that she grew up with went to a local amusement park; she always had loved roller coasters (a love I do not share), so we all went, and they rode until they were tired. It was great to see a genuine smile and hear that wonderful laugh again for a change. We spent one evening and the next morning there, and we all had a good time, not worrying about anything. She always had started doing some daily chores, but as winter had set in, getting outside very much was not an option. Still, we were once again enjoying our lives and were very thankful to be in the position we were in. We began to have a regular date night and started doing something that most of us neglect – we enjoyed the small things, thankful for each day and just the chance to be together. We would go out almost every Friday to see a movie then have a nice dinner; it was something small that we both looked forward to, and we were able to laugh and smile and just enjoy life. We made church a regular part of our lives, and I often think of how profound some of the messages I heard were and how they applied to our lives. One that sticks in my mind was the admonition to not "build bridges that you may never cross"; I did this a lot during the first month, and on many occasions since I imagined all the bad things that could happen and how I would deal with those things. In effect, in my mind I put myself through those things, and many of them never came to pass; they are burdens that may never be ours. We need to wait until we are at that crossing to build the bridge.

Behold the fowls of the air: for they sow not, neither do they reap, nor gather into barns; yet your heavenly Father feedeth them. Are ye not much better than they? (Mt 6:6)

Which of you by taking thought can add one cubit unto his stature? (Mt 6:27)

No matter how much we worry, or how good at it we are, it will never change anything, we cannot make ourselves any taller, healthier, richer or anything by worrying. As we continued to strive toward some since of normal, she continued to improve physically, but her short-term memory and her grasp of names and words was still an issue that seemed to stay with her, but we were happy to be alive and together. We were still aware of the prognosis, and it loomed over us always, but when you are in a fight you cannot spend all of your time thinking about when you got hit.

Winter gave way to spring, it was time to plant our crops and get on with our lives, I was starting to think that maybe I could get back to work soon, she had her three-month MRI around February after completing her radiation, and as always there is that fear, and the worry that we should not be doing, but it seemed to always accompany the post MRI doctors' appointments, and to our relief all went well. We began to think of our future again, to start planning and working toward our dreams that we were once again beginning to embrace. Then in May we returned for her next three-month scan. When visiting the doctor for our follow-up, we were told at that time that the tumor had begun to re-grow, we were once again crushed, just when it seemed that things were going to be OK, this. The doctor continued to explain that he would need to do a third surgery to resect as much of the tumor as possible; this would be three brain surgeries in nine months.

The ride home was very somber. We did not talk much. When we walked in the door, we fell in each other's arms and wept, again, but as with the chemo, Barbie was able to make the decision for herself. She spent time praying and talking to the Lord, and that was when she will tell you that she heard the Lord speak to her the second time, saying the same words, simply "Go ahead." She told me, "I am going to fight this and will not give up, I will have the surgery."

We also met with our radiologist who reviewed the scan and was adamant that what he was looking at was not tumor regrowth, he then sent us to Columbus, Ohio, for a PET scan, this was supposedly much more accurate a identifying tumors. This scan was completed, and it confirmed that it was tumor regrowing; again the doctor disputed the findings, but said, "At this point, I have no other option but to refer you to your surgeon." The call was made and surgery was scheduled for the first part of June, again. Barbie stepped up her exercise and began preparing for the next round of her battle. Again the darkness loomed thick over us. We spent a couple of days in a numb daze.

Friday rolled around, and Barbie said, "Where you taking me for our date?" She would continually refuse to let this take her life from her. Now you would think at this point one would start to think that the fight was over, but if so, you don't know Barbie, her resolve was strengthened and she was more determined than ever that this was a fight she would win, again that courage that never ceases to amaze me was on display, as the day approached she did not show fear, did not act nervous and seemed ready to face what was to come, she wasn't fooling anybody, I knew how she felt. I spent a lot of time in prayer and reading the Bible; this had become my preferred pastime while waiting in radiation waiting rooms, doctor offices, etc. I no longer felt far from God, but in need of his strength, one of the most valuable lessons, I have learned who was in control. There was a time when I thought I could tackle any problem and take care of it on my own. The day when you learn this is not the case is a sobering day, but what can follow is also a liberating day, the day you learn that he is in control and that you can let go.

Casting all your care upon him; for he careth for you. (1Pe 5:7)

This is profound: There is someone who you can say to "I can't handle this, would you please take it," and if we will let it go there is the peace that cannot be understood. In these times, you also realize when you stop relying on your own strength is when you can truly be strong.

And he said unto me, My grace is sufficient for thee: for my strength is made perfect in weakness. Most gladly therefore will I rather glory in my infirmities, that the power of Christ may rest upon me. (2Co 12:9)

As the surgery day drew closer, we talked about a lot of

things, we went and preformed the unpleased task of creating a living will, I would advise anyone who thinks they want one to do it while you are health, it's not a big deal then, but it is a very big deal when you are in a fight. It's kind of like bringing a stretcher in between rounds of a prize fight. And through it all, I did my best to keep my fears hidden, if she was not going to show hers, I would not try to drag it out of her, after all, her strength and faith was the one constant in our lives.

I spent time thinking about all the good things in our life, the fact that we loved each other and enjoyed spending time together, I thought of the things that we had already came through, drawing courage from past victories, doing everything that I could to make an attempt to match the courage that I knew would soon be on display very soon. We should be careful not to confuse courage and fear, anyone who would find their selves in this situation is going to experience fear, but courage is facing that fear and doing what the situation calls for. This is what I would witness – we would face our fears together, then we would face them alone when we were apart, then we would do what had to be done, and that was for my sweet wife to go in and have brain surgery number three. Yet even after two successful surgeries, it still struck fear in my heart.

Chapter 8
Days in the Sun

I've have written much about the good times that Barbie and I shared and the thought that because of our storm, the sun shines much brighter. We do have a great relationship and a great life, if not in spite of then because of Barbie's cancer. But the fact is that we all have our days when the sun shines but there are clouds scattered about in the bright skies, the challenge that we must face on those days with the scattered clouds, which is most days, is not to spend all of our times staring at the clouds. We can find ourselves much like kids trying to see what we can imagine in the shapes of the cloud, when we have an opportunity to enjoy the sun shining in our lives.

Through all of this, we have learned to enjoy small blessings and the day to day things that were always overlooked when we were young, healthy and busy – things like appreciating a good night's sleep and not getting out of bed hurting. There are many who would trade much for either of those. Or waking in a house, having something to eat, the ability to take a deep breath. None of these things should be taken for granted, but we all do. We go through many days surrounded by beauty, a wonderful sunrise, snow-covered trees, spring-time blooming trees, flowers, bluebird skies and the list could go on and on, but many times we are focused on the person driving in front of us that is too slow for us, or the bill that we need to pay, or maybe someone said something that we felt was mean to us, and we will miss the blessing and enjoyment of an otherwise great day.

A good example of this: I was driving home from working out of town one day, I was three or four hours from home, and I cut in front of a gentleman, kind of close. He almost came unglued, he made it a point to get ahead of me, cut close in front, honking his horn, hanging out his window, and yelling at me and gesturing that I am a number one driver. Now, I am not an overly timid person and do not shy from conflict as much as I should; I am, however, getting better and this day allowed me to come to a revelation that helped me greatly. I was getting upset when I thought to myself, "I sure am glad that I am not having as bad of a day as he is." I thought of how his day must be going if a little thing like that had set him off so severely. I said a little prayer of thanks giving that my day was not like his. I also said a prayer that his day would get better, I continued my drive home, thankful that I had not let his day rub off on me, I could have steamed all the way home and missed all the joy of a safe trip on a great day, with my wonderful wife waiting at the end of it. I could have let myself got so worked up on the way home that I ruined her day also when I got home, because our bad day, just like our good day, will rub off on those around us.

We have had many days in the sun since her diagnosis and grim prognosis, and we continue to experience them, but we look for them, we find them in a simple day when we both feel good and are able to be together, in a nice meal shared, fellowship with family and friends, a simple visit or phone conversation with our son always brings joy to us both, but a particularly wide smile to Barbie's face. Our weekly date night, when it can be taken, brings us both great joy in simple things, when she has taken chemo or radiation and we suspend our date in favor of staying away from crowd due to a weakened immune system, it makes them that much more enjoyable when we are able to resume them. A simple drive through the country talking about old times, now days I do most of the talking and she the listening, but the smile on her face as we travel the back roads speaks volumes. There is also great joy in a kind word from a neighbor or friend, or sharing a kind word with them, there are many who are going through trials much the same as us, and there is a wonderful blessing when you can lift someone else's day a little.

When we are lucky enough to be able to take a vacation, again we looked for the sunshine and found it in the small things a lot of times even when on a big trip. We stayed in a bed and breakfast on the banks of the Batten Kill River for a couple of days and very much enjoyed sitting around and talking to our host, one of whom had grown up just down the road from Norman Rockwell. He told us of stories from his youth of playing in the creek below so they could be in range to be the first available if help was needed, because the pay was better than mowing lawns. He let us see a painting that he posed for as a youth, he and I spent a morning fly fishing on the river while Barbie sat in the backyard and enjoyed watching the river flow by. Driving around on what we call "lost trips," we came across small New England towns with Revolutionary War museums and monuments. We toured those and and had a wonderful time .. On most of these trips we start out our day with no agenda; we just go looking for joy, and I have found that if that is what you are looking for, then that is what you find. On one such ride we saw a sign for maple syrup for sale; we stopped and ended up sitting on a picnic table with a wonderful lady for quite some time, just talking and getting to know each other. We traveled to Michigan to visit a good friend and his wife, both of who had experienced recurrences of long past cancers – his melanoma that had went to the brain and abdomen; hers breast cancer that had went to the bone. They were both in the fight, living and loving life as it came, he looking for another hunting season with friends and family, her, just enjoying family and taking care of him. Sometimes when you think you have it hard, you meet someone that makes you ashamed to feel sorry for yourself. Here they were both taking the role of patient and caregiver; I loved them both dearly. She since has went home to her reward, he is still in the fight looking for yet another deer season, but would be just as satisfied to go home to be with his love.

Many may wonder how that can be done with the shadow of a prognosis like theirs or Barbie's hanging over us, but we all have that prognosis, it's just that we have not been made aware of it.

A Psalm of David.
The LORD is my shepherd; I shall not want.
2 He maketh me to lie down in green pastures: he leadeth me beside the still waters.
3 He restoreth my soul: he leadeth me in the paths of righteousness for his name's sake.
4 Yea, though I walk through the valley of the shadow of death, I will fear no evil: for thou art with me; thy rod and thy staff they comfort me.
5 Thou preparest a table before me in the presence of mine enemies: thou anointest my head with oil; my cup runneth over.
6 Surely goodness and mercy shall follow me all the days of

my life: and I will dwell in the house of the LORD for ever. (Ps 23:1-6)

This is one of the most known chapters in the Bible and a source of much comfort. I have heard speculation on the location of the valley of the shadow of death, I have heard preachers talk about its location somewhere in the Middle East, but it is not that hard, the valley of the shadow of death is life, from the day we are born, death haunts our footsteps and hangs over us like a shadow, death is a part of life just like birth is. Most do not like to hear this, but after you accept it and get over it, then you can take the comfort and blessing out of these verses, for we are not in this valley alone. When we accept that death is just a part of life,the sting is gone and the valley is a little less dark.

Yes, healthy or sick learn to take joy from the small things, like a sunrise or a sunset, make an effort to enjoy these in a special place if the opportunity avails itself. Make time to visit a close friend and catch up, there may not be another chance. This brings to mind that we should not let things go unsaid; we will have sadness at the loss of a loved one, but we can make sure that we do not have regrets over things left unsaid, say the, I love you, the I'm sorry, the I forgive you. Do not let an event that we all know is coming take you by surprise and leave you with a life time of regret that can never be addressed, this is something else you face when you think you know it is coming soon. I have to smile when I think of all the times that I thought I knew what God was doing in our lives just to find out that I was not even close, you would think after several times I would stop thinking that I know, and making plans around what I think I know, you would be wrong. For some reason the lessons taught are far more than the lessons learned, or maybe just the lessons practiced.

Wherefore seeing we also are compassed about with so great a cloud of witnesses, let us lay aside every weight, and the sin which doth so easily beset us, and let us run with patience the race that is set before us... (Heb 12:1)

I find the challenge of putting aside my weights easier than in times past; the challenge I find is to leave them alone and not pick them back up. The good thing is He did not say we could only cast our burdens on Him once, He will take them back. This is the only way I have found to face the storms with peace in my heart.

Peace I leave with you, my peace I give unto you: not as the world giveth, give I unto you. Let not your heart be troubled, neither let it be afraid. (Joh 14:27)

To enjoy the small things is another lesson I've learned. Sometimes there is a big thing that we have to get out of our way. I know that if you are in the middle of a storm now that may seem impossible to do. We know; we have been there. It takes time. You have read of many tears shed, many miles walked in sadness, many sleepless nights, all these were on the road to acceptance of our circumstance, the road to finding the joy in our lives. I have given a lot of advice that at this time may seem out of reach if you are looking into the darkness, but we want to give you hope, the light will shine again, the hope of this chapter is that you stop and look, it may be shining now and you just cannot see it yet, it is even more important to enjoy the day if you may have less of them. Do not let cancer or any other life-threatening disease take your joy from you. You may not be able change the avenue by which you meet your appointment with death, but your joy is yours to control.

1 In the beginning was the Word, and the Word was with God, and the Word was God.

2 The same was in the beginning with God.

3 All things were made by him; and without him was not any thing made that was made.

4 In him was life; and the life was the light of men.

5 And the light shineth in darkness; and the darkness comprehended it not.

6 There was a man sent from God, whose name was John.

7 The same came for a witness, to bear witness of the Light, that all men through him might believe.

8 He was not that Light, but was sent to bear witness of that Light.

9 That was the true Light, which lighteth every man that cometh into the world.

10 He was in the world, and the world was made by him, and the world knew him not.

11 He came unto his own, and his own received him not.

12 But as many as received him, to them gave he power to become the sons of God, even to them that believe on his name:

13 Which were born, not of blood, nor of the will of the flesh, nor of the will of man, but of God.

14 And the Word was made flesh, and dwelt among us, (and we beheld his glory, the glory as of the only begotten of the Father,) full of grace and truth. (Joh 1-14)

I have included many passages from Scripture and written

a lot of faith, but my goal is to help a fellow traveler who finds himself surround by darkness. I only know the way that we made it through and still are able to live a blessed life, even in the valley of the shadow of death.

When I think about our days in the sun, it brings a smile to my face, lazy days floating on lake fishing, traveling to watch or favorite college basketball team, and Barbie's habit of rooting for the team that has the ball. I think of walks shared in the country just enjoying each other's company, the countless laughs shared and the smile that can brighten my day. I look back with much joy and am happy that we made the decision to enjoy our lives while we have them, there has been much joy that could have been taken from us if we had let that happen.

Chapter 9
Surgery No. 3,
The Clouds Part

Once again we were preparing for what seemed to me as the impossible, a third brain surgery. The surgery itself was still a scary thing – after all it is brain surgery – but it was not as scary as the first time. The thing that occupied my thoughts and drove my fears was the fact that just a few short months after her last two surgeries and radiation the cancer was back. Was the grim prognosis correct? Did we have only a short time left together here in this earth? Again the bridge crew was out building those bridges that I may or may not have to cross, even though I knew better. We are like that, even the strongest. The Apostle Paul said that he did the things he knew not to do and did not the things he knew that he should. So now that is where I find myself, but again Barbie is the picture of courage, the absolute bravest person I have ever met, when I should have been her strength, Whether she knew it or not, she was mine.

When the day arrived for the surgery, Barbie again walked into arena like a gladiator, but this time with a clear understanding that we were coming back to be with her in pre-op. We gathered early; I probably have not expressed enough how grateful I am for having a wonderful family, friends, church and community. When I talked to each, I always could relay how things were going, tell them of Barbie's condition and be steady, but when the offers of help and the expression of love came, the lump in my through always stopped my speech. This journey would be so difficult without The Lord and each of the aforementioned, so once again, I want to express my deepest gratitude to all those who care and those who stand beside me.

We all gathered around her in the pre-op and surrounded her with love until they wheeled her off. I can never forget the feeling of watching her go down the hall and out of sight – a view of helplessness, loneliness, and desperation. Then the long wait began, again. My thoughts drifted to the *what ifs*, the *what will I do's*. Much time was spent in prayer. The hours slowly crawled by. I thought of the lady I had heard on television talked about her fight with breast cancer, and how her attitude had helped us. She spoke of the *why me* stage that I think all are faced with when going through crises, and how one day it came to her, "Why not me?" When you think about it, "Why me?" implies that someone else is more deserving of what you are going through than you. It's not about deserving, though, it's just about life. There is an element of comfort when you get past the thought that what you are going through was sent just for you. When you get past that, then you can look to those who have experienced the same – and yes others have – and you can draw on their trials and more importantly, their victories for your help. By this time, I had read a lot online about the disease that Barbie was in the grips of; I did know that there were survivor stories but still the worry that it had returned so soon drove my fears.

The day wore on with no word from the operating room.

One hour turned into two and two to three, then about four or five hours into the surgery, word came from the operating room that it seemed that all that was being removed was scar tissue. My heart leapt at this glimmer of hope. Of course, there was still more to be done and things could change, but for now we had some good news, and that has been a scarce commodity. I was struck by the fact that when going through times like these how even the smallest hope is still hope, and how one will grasp for it, and cling to it. Do not think that the small bit of help that you can give someone who is going through hard time is not enough to help. It all helps – the phone calls, the visits, the kind words spoken with sincerity – they all contribute to lifting the spirit a little, and a little lift always is very appreciated.

Finally the doctor comes out to speak with us, he does confirm that all that he found was scar tissue, that he had removed it, and that she was doing very well. We were all very relieved, hugs were exchanged, prayers of thanksgiving were given, and family and friends started drifting out once again. Soon we were left with just the closest of family to wait until we could see her. We sat around and talked, often bringing up the good news and how that maybe all was going to be OK; after all, the wait seemed much shorter than in previous surgeries. For the first time while sitting in the hospital, I allowed myself to dream of our future. I built bridges to good places, thought about our house that we would build, our son's graduation, family vacations, and in all of these thoughts, she was there. It had been a while since I had allowed myself these thoughts, and it hit me that even when being positive, that thoughts of a negative outcome still were there.

Upon entering the ICU, I was greeted with a much too familiar sight – my lovely wife, hooked to monitors with tubes coming out of her head, which was completely wrapped in bandages, lying unconscious in her bed. The joy and relief I had felt earlier was hard to lay hold on now, as I sat by her bed, continuing to reflect on our lives, our dreams, our hopes. Then at the sound of a monitor I would be snapped back to our reality. I knew that it would be another long healing process, there would be weeks of total care needed, months of watchfulness. I relished the role of caregiver; it was what I wanted to do and what she needed from me at this time. I reflected on the vows we had taken on our wedding day and how we had talked prior to that day. I had told her if we did not mean each and every one of them, then we should not take them, I take them serious, I vowed a vow to her before God, and I intended to keep them, it seems that now as I look back we have been in each of the situations we addressed when we took them.

The recovery went well once again;I allowed myself to hope that Barbie had come through this surgery better than any of the rest. We stopped by the drugstore and got prescriptions filled and made the journey home. She again was in that familiar post-surgery fog. At home, I resumed my role as chief caregiver, a roll that I had never imagined myself in and had not wanted, but was thankful for that I was there and had the ability to do what needed to be done. After her first surgery, watermelon was the only thing that she seemed to want to eat. The second surgery it was mashed potatoes and gravy from one of the fried chicken restaurants, many hour-long round trips were made to satisfy her craving. This time she seemed to be more accepting of what was fixed, but sausage biscuits and gravy were always a hit. That was a good thing, as this is one of my specialties. One morning that

I was fixing that for breakfast, my boss stopped by to check on us and bring a collection that was taken up by my co-workers. I thanked him, but he told me he was only the delivery boy, and that it had all been done by friends I worked with. We have been truly blessed to live and work in areas that people still reach out to each other in times of need. He ask how things had been going and how Barbie was getting along. We all visited for a while; he told me that he and most of my co-workers had changed companies (a common event in my field of employment) and that when I got ready to return to let him know. I told him that I hoped that would be possible, but it was too early to know at this time, he agreed and sincerely wished me the best and made the offer that always chokes me up, "If you need anything..."

As the days progressed, Barbie's recovery went well; she had indeed came out of this surgery better than either of the last two. She could converse much better, and while there were still issues with short-term memory, names came better than before, as did the words she was looking for when speaking. She still had an issue with fatigue, that seemed to be harder to recover from than first thought, but all in all she was much better than I had hoped.

The first two of the three month MRIs came and went with no issues, and we had hope that maybe the clouds were lift-ing and life or some semblance of the life we had known could return. We still considered all the sickness and treat-ments that we had been through as terrible times in our lives; at that time, not enough of life had passed to see that maybe it was not as dark as what we were seeing.we found it to be very hard not to look at the clouds when you are in the storm, but there is one who see through the storm and knows what is on the other side.

Declaring the end from the beginning, and from ancient times the things that are not yet done, saying, My counsel shall stand, and I will do all my pleasure... (Isa 46:10)

Many times in my life, I have looked back on the bad times and realized that they were just the path that I had to walk to get to the good.

As time passed, Barbie regained her ability to work around the house, cook, clean and her position as chief homemaker. Her ability to work outside the house at public jobs was negativity affected by her short-term memory loss, but that was OK. As she continued to take responsibilities that I had assumed, and began to care for herself and our young son, the time had come for me to get back to work. I contacted my old boss with his new company, and with the company I was working with when she got sick, and let them know I wanted to come back to work; the only stipulation was that I could no longer be a contractor – I had to have a position with health insurance. I had learned my lesson. During this time, another company had heard that I was looking for a job and contacted me also, so interviews were set up with all three companies. As I met with each, and as with all interviews since that day, I first lay out Barbie's condition and explain where my priorities will be if she needs me. After all the interviews were completed, I was offered a position with all three companies. I chose to go with the company that my old boss and all of my previous co-workers who had reached out so generously to me were at. My new role was a step below supervision but came with a steady salary and full benefit package. We were very happy and things were looking up, Barbie was doing very well, able to do most of the things she wanted to do, and thankful for the health that she had. The things that were lost were not the issue; the things, including the life that she had, was what we focused on, and in that we started to appreciate things more that we had in the past taken for granted.

Another MRI came and went, and the three month schedule was moved to six months. I once again found myself traveling on my job and spending time on the road in motels. Barbie and I would talk every morning and every evening. She was taking care of the home and our son, I was earning a living, and we were farming; in short, life was getting back to normal. We tried to never fail to be thankful for what we had and the blessings we received. Life always includes the good and the bad; we choose what we focus on. One thing that had struck us both along our journey was how many people were going through much the same – and many times worse things – than we were. You do not notice until you are thrust into that place. We noticed the many young people, that short of a miracle, never would see the age we had reached, and that madefeeling sorry for ourselves much harder. It had been a very eye-opening experience, and though the statementeems strange to say, not all bad.

After reading some of Barbie's journals, I realized how much she was fighting fatigue during this time. She struggled with issues raising our teenage son while I was on the road, running to do chores, and keeping the house up, so she was tired most of the time but did not tell anyone, just continued doing what had to be done as she always had. She also took on the job of a contract loss adjuster. She would be dealing with local farmers, working their claims. I would help with paperwork and she, after some training, did the field work. She had rode along for years with me on claims, so she had a good feel for the job. All of the farmers either already knew her or quickly got to; she did very well, but again, it added to her fatigue. Many of her journal entries ended with "I am tired now, going to try to lay down a little while."

Around this time, I received a promotion into supervision at my job, which came with a nice pay raise. The six-month MRIs came and went, and we finally arranged to pour the walls for our house. It had been a long journey, after her first surgery the wall of the hole for the basement had collapsed, and we had them cleaned out later after her second surgery, then when we found out about her third to come, we again delayed and one wall collapsed again, so this time we cleaned it out and poured our walls. It had been so long, and with the money on hand we made the decision to use our logs as beam work and build a underground house with a peak roof and cathedral ceiling. So the log cabin was abandoned in favor of getting into our new place sooner. My brother, who was a contractor at the time, built our house on my design, and before you know it (though at the time it did not seem that quick), we were moving in. By the time we moved in up, the fatigue had built to the point that I did not want Barbie working in the fields anymore, and dad was at the age where he did not need a lot to do, so I signed most of the farm up in a set-aside program, leaving just enough to raise feed for the cattle, so it has turned into more of a hobby, and my job into more of a job, we are continually blessed and my salary exceeded expectations. As I got busier I found the time to help Barbie complete or double-check her paperwork was no longer there, she eventually let her adjusting job go also. More six-month MRIs came and went without any problems, and they were moved out to a yearly schedule. We have been able to take vacations, just as the doctor once ordered; we had been blessed to spend time in the winter on the Southern coast for meetings that we extended into vacations. I have a picture on my computer of a time in the Everglades when I was surprised by Barbie saying, "Hey Dave." I turned to find her holding a baby alligator that was about two and a half feet long. We have spent time several summers in the Northeast, mountains and East Coast, and since our son has grown Barbie has taken to traveling with me much of the time. The supervisor position involved working at home a lot, and we are getting back the time we lost when I had to travel all the time. We continued to count our blessings as the yearly MRIs came and went. In what seemed to be no time, five years had passed with no problem. We were living a wonderful life, we loved our home on the hill, we were able to pay off our home and have been blessed beyond belief. After she got sick and she got saved, and I rededicated my life to the Lord or life has been happier than we could have ever imagined it would be. And now we can both look back and see that the storm was not all bad, just as actual storms come, lightning flashes, wind blows, and thunder rolls, often there is damage done, but the rain arrives and waters the ground, and things grow and the good comes.

During that time, a friend and I started making yearly, week-long bow hunting trips. About a month prior to one of these trips, I had been feeling a little ill, and as I am prone to do, I ignored the symptoms until in the middle of the night I was hit with an abdominal pain that doubled me over and pushed me very near to passing out. I made it back to bed and lay down, then woke up Barbie and told her that I needed to go to the hospital. She was understandable panicked; I had to ask her to slow down a couple of times, as the rough spots in the road were very painful. After arriving, it was determined that my appendix had ruptured, emergency surgery was scheduled, and Barbie found herself on the other side of the bed. She was very distressed. I have been blessed with good health, and this was out of her element, but she rose to the challenge and became my caregiver. I recovered quickly, and in two weeks got permission from the doctor to go on my hunting trip, which I did. Now this was not my wisest decision, and I would advise anyone who is thinking about a hunting trip less than a month after major surgery, don't. I made it and all went OK, but it was not nearly as fun as the rest had been, and Barbie was put through extra worry back home.

Chapter 10
A Normal Life

Life continued along much like everyone else's, and we had many long talks about the road we walked, how that even in the worst things there is good. Many people who we had once counted as friends, that were on the previous path that we were on had passed away from one thing or another, and as we talked, many times after attening funerals, we wondered where we might be had we not changed our path. We pondered on the possibility that what seemed to be a prognosis that would shorten Barbie's life, could have been the vehicle by which both or either of our lives may have been lengthened, it is something that can neer be known, but what we do know is we are very happy on the path that we are on. When people who love each other face things like this, one of two things can happen – they can fall apart or they will draw closer than most people can imagine. That has been the result in our lives; we have a relationship that most never will experience and regardless of the length of it, I would not trade it for anything. The following is an entry that was made into Barbie's journal in 2003:

> *Dear Lord; I want to thank you for everything you have given me, the best and the worst, because it has made my life wonderful and frightful, but also a great gift of eternal hope*

and a great Lord, Amen.

The experience is reflected in every aspect of our lives, at my work, my peers sometimes cannot understand how I can face with such calm what they perceive as problems. I often tell them that what we are dealing with is not a problem, that I have seen problems, and they do not look like this. What we experience most of the time and approach as a problem is just a situation that we have to deal with; it may take more time or special attention, but in the end, no matter the outcome, life will go on tomorrow as normal. The experience has actually given me the ability to do much more efficiently the job that was asked. I always have been blessed with the ability to deal with people; this was enhanced by the lessons I have learned on the importance of listening. Many issues can be resolved with ease if we will take the time to listen, not just waiting on our turn to talk, but listening with some empathy and understanding.

The yearly MRIs continued to come and go with no issues, and life was good. I received a promotion to a manager's position and between working at home and traveling together, we are able to spend most of our time together, we are blessed to see much of our wonderful country traveling for work. We also have made many wonderful friends – who are more like family – through my work. During this time Barbie developed a curious habit of counting things as we travel, even from time to time using a pad and pen to keep track – red trucks, flags, ponds, recording license plates from different states. I am not sure where that came from, but it kept her amused for many miles. Traveling much like many other things wears her out, but she says it is better than staying home alone. That was something that has never bothered her. She would stay home at our hilltop, no outside lights and no neighbors, watching horror movies all evening. She has never relayed any time that she felt fear in the many nights of holding down the fort. Just another instance of her ability to adapt and do what is needed, and always with joy in her heart. She was happy at home taking care of what needed to be done and is happy traveling. I guess a girl has to do what a girl has to do also.

As we traveled, one constant has been Barbie's outgoing personality and lack of inhibitions, walking up to presidents and CEOs of very large nationwide companies, holding out her hand and saying "Hello, I'm Barbie." I remember the time she called the COO of my company a liar; we had just put on a training for a company that by boss and I had just recently joined, we had redone their entire training material and completely changed it from what had been done in the past; the COO had attended because of our change. The meeting had been a complete success, and she had offered to by us a drink. I do not drink but said that I would join them for a cup of coffee. As we sat for a while, Barbie came down from the room looking for me and meeting the chief officer in the hallway, she asked, "Have you seen Dave?" and was told that I was in the bar, to which Barbie replied, "You lie." A little put back, the lady replied, "No, he is drinking coffee." Her straightforward blunt speaking was always accompanied by much politeness and always referring to people as "young man" or "young lady," she always has been very well liked by all of my coworkers, bosses and most who have the pleasure of meeting her, but you seldom leave wondering what is on her mind.

Right around the time we got to move into our new house, we lost our two oldest golden retrievers, an event that was very hard on Barbie. She cried her eyes out, and even years after, she will still tear up when talking about them. They were very much family. I think of one time when we were off in town and heavy rains came, we had a new litter of eleven puppies, they and the female were locked in a small building we used to process tobacco in the winter. As the rains came, we had a flash flood and the water came up and got into the building, when we returned home, she was in a panic thinking the puppies may have drowned, but my brother and his son who lived next door had waded the water and rescued mother and all puppies. They were the heroes of the day. The litters of pups were a source of great joy; if I wanted to see her when they were young, I knew where to find her, and we had three liters then let our beloved female retire.

The last litter we had we agreed that we would keep one of the pups for our own; I explained to Barbie that we did not want to pick our puppy as soon as they were born but wanted to watch them for a while and pick one based on personality and attentiveness to us. The big day came while I was out working, and when one of the puppies was born, the umbilical cord would not stop bleeding, Barbie tied it off and put some medicine on it. When I got home, the puppies were about four hours old and ours was picked out. "I saved her life, this one is mine," she said. Baby animals have always held a spot in her heart, so springtime on the farm is a special time; when the weather begins to warm, it is a great pleasure looking out the windows at the baby calves running and jumping around the pasture. Over the years, the farm has afforded Barbie the opportunity to raise a multitude of baby animals – chickens, ducks, goats. She even had a special little angora goat named Rambo that was born to a goat we had bought, it was very pretty and she really loved it. Unfortunately, it was crossing the road one day and was hit by a car; it was a sad time for a while. There was the baby fawn that I caught while mowing hay, it had stood up and walked over into the tall hay and laid back down, sure to be killed by the mowing machine. I stopped the tractor and walked over and picked it up. We took it down to the barn at our house, and Barbie rubbed the fuzz off of it all day long. That evening we took it up and laid it back in the cut hay field where it had been before the hay was cut, we backed off and watched. Just before dark the doe came out and got it and they walked off into the woods. My girl had a smile that would not stop that evening. She had the pleasure of feeding orphaned baby calves with a bottle, said that reminded her of a time when she was little and a chicken hawk dropped a baby ground hog in their yard; she got it and fed it with an eye dropper, the ground hog survived, and she raised it to become the family pet. It lived in the house for years and was one of her beloved childhood pets. It seems she was always trying to save some kind of baby wild thing. There even was an attempt to save baby opossums found hanging on a road-killed mother, this was an unsuccessful attempt, but she tried. I am still not sure if she fell in love with me, or the farm and all of the animals roaming its hills. No matter – I am the one who is the richer for it.

This was typical of the little girl who grew up on her beloved Greasy Ridge. She was the oldest child of two. Growing up, her heroes were her dad whose shoulders she loved to ride around on as a little girl; he worked construction – she eagerly awaited his return when he was off working, always a surprise hidden in a pocket somewhere – and her Grandpa – a plain-spoken Baptist preacher who was also an equipment operator at a local gravel quarry (which actually adjoined our farm). her grandparents owned a small hilltop farm just out the ridge to the west from Barbie's parents, to which as she got older she would often walk out and play with the animals, and help out where she could, often picking black and red raspberries; she was often accused of eating more than she put into the bucket, an accusation that probably had some merit. She was often in trouble with her mother who liked to dress her little girl in pretty frilly dresses, which did not go well with the little girl who liked to play in the dirt and mud. This was the case one day when her two cousins who lived in the local town came out to visit, as they roamed around. Barbie thought it would be funny to bombard them with dried (or partially dried) horse droppings. It seemed to be a lot of fun for one of them, as the girls ran home screaming and gagging. She followed, I am sure with a gleeful laugh, until she got home, though when she tells the story I get the feeling that it was worth it.

As she grew older, she often earned extra money by working at the local farms with her cousin who lived just down the road. She could often be found hoeing or harvesting tobacco, or doing other odd jobs that they could find. In the fall, she would work at the local fairs while the family was in town. Around that time, her father injured his back in a work accident and was no longer able to work. This was also the time when she and her mother begin to have problems. Barbie was always a very strong-willed person, and apparently her mother was also. This led to many conflicts, after one of which she moved in with her aunt in town for a time. She bounced between there and home for a while as the conflict increased. Looking for a way out of the conflict led her to get married as soon as she was of age, and she moved off, but this eventually evolved into a relationship much like the one she had left.

When we met her life had been very tumultuous for the last fifteen years or so, a long time for a girl of the age of twenty-four. I have been blessed with a wonderful loving family, and upon meeting them all, Barbie compared them to a Seventies sitcom family, they all instantly took to Barbie and brought her into the loving fold of our family, something that had been missing for a long time in her life. She soon was calling my parents "mom and dad," and they had another daughter, as expressed below from her journal entry in 2004:

> It's Thanksgiving Day, I haven't wrote in my journal for a while, I've thought about it but I did not do it. I feel thankful for everything in my life, my life feels happier, stable fully loved by my husband, full of love and faith by the Lord. I feel great about my life, and I hope I'm living it as the Lord wants me to, I love all of my in-laws, but I love Mom and Dad the most, I love my son forever, my family I love. I hope one day I'll see Mom or Dad would through the Church doors, I guess that's the Lords and their choice. Thank you everyone for being full of love and devotion for our family, I love you all forever.

One of the joys of my life has been seeing her reaction to being surrounded by love, and the joy it has brought her. My sister later told me with some sorrow in her voice that after we got married that she was a little jealous of Barbie. My sister had moved off of the farm to work in a hospital, and Barbie was here, calling our parents "Mom" and "Dad." My sister said that she felt bad for this; we told her not to, because people that love each other as we do always get past that.

The years continued to roll by, and before we thought it possible, we were going in for the ten year MRI and neurologist visit. A decade had passed; that was hard to comprehend. Everything was good, and yearly MRIs were discontinued, though we did keep seeing the neurologist to maintain the seizure pills that she was taking and would probably be on for the rest of her life. This was such a blessing, but also a little surreal. Ten years ago, she was told that she only had six months to live, but she took up the fight with a determination that was awe-inspiring. The Lord had taught us a lesson about thinking that we knew what he had planned for our lives. Instead of being separated after six months, we had just completed living ten of the happiest years that anyone could have experienced. I thank God every day, for my wonderful wife and the time he has allowed us.

7 Ask, and it shall be given you; seek, and ye shall find; knock, and it shall be opened unto you:

8 For every one that asketh receiveth; and he that seeketh findeth; and to him that knocketh it shall be opened.

9 Or what man is there of you, whom if his son ask bread, will he give him a stone?

10 Or if he ask a fish, will he give him a serpent?

11 If ye then, being evil, know how to give good gifts unto your children, how much more shall your Father which is in heaven give good things to them that ask him? (Mt 7:7-11)

We had been so long going through regularly scheduled appointments with all good results and the MRIs had not been bad, but even with everything going good, there was a stress that had to be faced every time we would walk into the office to get the results of another scan. We felt a great since of relief when we heard that we would no longer need to endure that on a yearly basis.

Life continued to march on, and it was great. Sure, we had the everyday problems that everyone faces – medical issues with aging parents, a teenage son growing up, work, etc., you know, the normal things. *Normal*...what a great word.

We started taking yearly vacations, just the two of us. One morning on the coast of Maine, Barbie (who had always had a fear of deep water) surprised me by asking if I wanted to take the whale watching trip. I said, "You know we will go out past sight of the shore?" She said, "Yes, let's try it." We had a great time. She started out sitting inside while the boat was under way but finished riding out on the front with the wind blowing her long hair. Maine was one of our favorite vacation destinations; we both like lobster, though Barbie liked them less after she opened her first fresh lobster and got a look inside; she ate a lot of shrimp and scallops on that trip! We ascended the Mt. Washington auto road; she was very quiet and glad when that one was over, as the narrow road and steep drop offs plummeting thousands of feet, were not to her liking. Had I not been watching the road so close, I am sure I would have seen her eyes closed.

We also watched the sun rise over the Grand Canyon, something that we both agreed was one of the most beautiful things we had witnessed. Sitting there before daybreak with the one you love, awaiting the sunrise, and then marveling as the gray and darkness gave way to brilliant colors, watching as the darkness of the canyon slowly gave way as the sun made its way deeper and deeper into the canyon was something That we found breath taking, a memory we will both cherish all of our days. She flew for the first time ever on that trip. I watched over and over as she faced fears and displayed the courage I had come to be in awe of.

We have explored several mountain ranges and find that we enjoy them more than we do beaches. Once we rented a cabin in a small Vermont mountain resort with nothing around other that small mom-and-pop stores, we spent days just sitting on the porch, cooking out and enjoying our surroundings. We explored caves when the opportunity presented itself – no spelunking, just guided tours, but this we also found very enjoyable. We also had many adventures on work outings during this time. We got to take a airboat tour of the Everglades, stern wheel rides with shows and dinners on the Mississippi at a couple of different locations, a tour of a historical flour milling operation at the Mississippi headwaters, and several beachfront winter meetings. The one thing that always seemed to come through was that it seemed to not take a lot to entertain a couple of hillbillies.

The next five years continued to roll by at a very relaxed and enjoyable pace. The loans were getting paid off, the everyday stresses that we all face when we were younger were subsiding, and we never ceased to give thanks. Barbie teaches children's Sunday school, which is something she really enjoys because it lets her interact with young ones, and I have taken the position of adult Sunday school teacher in our church. The Lord had truly blessed us both.

But many times the good thing and times of this life, just like the bad, do not last forever, this wonderful stretch of blessed living has now lasted for fifteen years...fifteen years since she received the six month prognosis, fifteen years of a wonderful life surrounded by love and a marriage that most will never experience, a time when all arguments could be counted on one hand and have fingers to spare. It's a normal Sunday morning, and we are getting ready for Church.

Chapter 11
Our Faith Tested

A couple of months before that Sunday we first started to notice something...some words were getting hard to find, at first not anything that most people would notice, only your closest friend. As the days passed, the concern mounted steadily after fifteen years we did not have to worry anymore. An upcoming yearly visit with the neur ologist already scheduled in a couple of weeks, so we just waited. During the visit, it was mentioned that we had noticed some difficulty, a few simple word finding test were performed, and The Doctor decided that an MRI would be in order. There was a little concern, but she went in for the test and we went home; no doctor appointment had been made. Then the call came from the surgeon who we had not seen for over a decade –"We need you to come in and discuss your MRI." Our hearts dropped, we had no doubt now what that meant, but we tried to be strong for each other, each trying to fool the other. We went about our lives as if nothing was up for the next few days until the appointment day arrived.

At last, we went in to see the doctor who had been instrumental in saving her life a decade and a half ago. His message was short and blunt: It's back and there is nothing that I can do, but you have had a good run. We were taken completely off guard; I had been warned that the doctor was not like he used to be, and for quite some time I felt very angry at him for this delivery that left absolutely no hope. After some thought, I realized that a lifetime of delivering bad news, helping patients last a little longer, and them seeing them pass must take a horrific toll on a person, and he had been great when we needed him; this did not change the past. But those thoughts did not come that day. That day, the darkness set back in, the tears returned, but it was not the same as before, the hard phone calls to family were placed, and we began to let reality set in. We were referred to a new surgeon who was practicing in the hospital, a bright young man with amazing bedside manner and a glowing positive personality, just who we needed at that time. He told us that the location was inoperable, but that did not mean that it was untreatable. The tumors – yes *plural* – were small, and The decision was made that waiting a couple months and doing another MRI would be the best course for now, then there were a couple of treatment options available. We did meet with our radiologist who told us that radiation was not an options as the area had received the maximum radiation that was allowable already. After the news had a few days to sink in, we slowly began to try to resume a since of normal in our lives, we had long ago decided that no one knows when their last day is, and we did not want to waste days worrying about when one of ours would be, we try to live each day as it comes, and be thankful when the next one rolls around.

1 Cast thy bread upon the waters: for thou shalt find it after many days

2 Give a portion to seven, and also to eight; for thou knowest not what evil shall be upon the earth.

3 If the clouds be full of rain, they empty themselves upon the earth: and if the tree fall toward the south, or toward the

93

north, in the place where the tree falleth, there it shall be.

4 He that observeth the wind shall not sow; and he that regardeth the clouds shall not reap. (Ec 11:1-4)

We have realized that life goes on, even in the storm, with or without us, we can chose to live, love and enjoy what we have, or cry moan and be miserable, so life went on. During this time, we took one of our most enjoyable vacations to date – we flew out to California and rented a large SUV, and then we drove back across the beautiful country to Ohio. The first stop we made was in the Sequoia National Park, we marveled at the trees and took many pictures .Barbie was in awe, I had been there when I was young, but she had only seen the trees on TV; her reaction was worth all the effort to get there. Our next memorable stop was the Grand Canyon. As stated earlier, were amazed. We worked our way on home, stopping where we wanted, we visited a good friend in the Ozarks, and then made our way home. During that time, we gave no thought to our dilemma, we just enjoyed out time together and the opportunity we had. It's worth saying again – we have the choice, life will go on, we can live it and enjoy the day we have, or let our circumstance take the joy from the days we have. We may be worrying about only having a few months, when in reality we could not have tomorrow.

After we got home, we started looked into new treatments, trials and the searching for hope that one does when faced with this dilemma. Barbie still felt well, and aside from the issue with finding some words, everything was the same. Then came that Sunday. She had taken her shower and was looking for something to fix for breakfast, I heard her rummage through the cabinets as I got into the shower. When I got out, I glanced into the living room and saw her sitting on the couch reading a package of oats. I dressed and came out; she was still in the same position and not moving, just sitting straight up on the couch, holding the package up in front of her face. I "woke" her up and when she came to, she could not talk and was very confused. We got ready and headed to the emergency room. Thoughts raced through my head, I started building those bridges again...Would she come out of it? Had I heard her sweet voice for the last time? Would she get worse? All these thoughts rattling around in my head, as I drove in silence. As we got closer to town, I called my parents and let them know what was going on and told them to go ahead and go to church. She seemed to feel fine and actually be doing fine, words just would not come. After about an hour in the emergency room, she spoke a couple of words, and within another half hour she was talking and feeling good, She lost some use of her right arm and was left with weakness in her right leg. As days went on, that would lead to a lot of falls and leave her too weak to get up on her own. The storm clouds were gathering once again.

Shortly after returning home, the reality set in – she would not be able to stay alone, at least for a while. I had to help her up and steady her as she walked, I would need to take on all of the homemaking task along with being her caregiver and earning a living. We were no longer left with the option of not working, the health care I had insisted on fifteen years earlier would now be the avenue to her treatment. Just as all of this was happening, the company that I worked for was sold, in a very competitive industry. Relationships are highly valued, and over the last few years I had developed many good ones, so when word got out of the sale, I soon had a couple of options as to where I would work. I was truly blessed, especially when you consider that I have never attended college; I learned my craft on the job. So during the first three or four months of her ordeal, work was not an issue; we were just finishing things up and awaiting the transition, and I was able to stay at home. I then sat down with the upper management from the company that had purchased ours; I went into great detail about Barbie's tumor and treatment and the fact that I may have to work only from home for a while. They made a very good offer. In the meantime, my boss who I had worked with for close to twenty years took a position with another company, and he asked if I would interview with them. I agreed. In this interview, I sat down with the president of the company and was very taken with his business philosophies and the value he placed on integrity, honesty and family. Again I spoke at length about Barbie and what was going on; she accompanied me on that trip, and they were able to meet. The offer was not as good, but it felt to me that this was the place I was to be. After many days spent in prayer and trying to get a feel for what was right for me, the money difference was significant, but I just kept coming back to the company that had offered less, so I followed what I took as the Lord's guidance.

In the following days, we visited with surgeons, a radiologist, and an oncologist. After weighing the options the decision was made that she would start on a chemo drug called Temodar; it was generally well tolerated and had shown to be effective against her type of tumor. She started on the drug and did not have a lot of issues, just some nausea that we learned to control. She was very tired and weak, which on top of the effects of her seizure left her unable to walk for any distance; we got her a wheelchair and would go to a local lake many days. We would walk together for as long as she could then I would push her along trails, trying to get out of the house as much as possible. Many days, we would take long rides along country roads after she had taken her dose of medicine, which was in pill form. We would ride around many of the same places that we did when we were dating, we would talk and laugh about the old times and our fond memories. We stopped up a dead end hollow one day and reminisced about our first date, where I had a flat tire on my truck; I told her that I always went the extra mile, most guys just ran out of gas. We spent many hours driving through the country that fall during each course of chemo, which lasted five days than twenty one days between doses; I very much enjoyed being able to spend time with her away from phones, computers and televisions. We again found joy in small things.

After three months, there was the first follow-up MRI, showing that the tumor was shrinking. During the visit with our neurologist, I ask if physical therapy would help her leg; his response was "I don't know, but it won't hurt," so we started three days a week physical therapy, and it did help a great deal. She started being able to walk longer distances, but still had some balance issues. Her arm also got a little better. My work has been great; during interviews I always make sure to talk about her condition and stress that if she needs me I will be with her, and if that would not be acceptable, don't hire me. I was allowed to work mostly from home, the few meetings I did have to attend she would go with me, and just as had been happening at home, it was not unusual to come in and find her on the floor. I felt so bad for her; she had worked and fought so hard. As had always been the case, there was no feeling sorry for herself, and it seemed that she had a difficult time grasping that she could not do something. Many of her falls stemmed from her lack of inhibitions, as realizing that something was not a good idea did not happen. For instance, there was the day in Overland Park, Kansas, that I was at a meeting about a half mile from the motel. I told her I would be back at lunch and bring us something. She had looked out at the restaurant that was about a quarter mile away and decided to walk over and get some lunch. She fell at the door of the motel, Two of the maids helped her up and got her into her room, then they went and got her a drink to replace the one she had spilled. When I got back, I could tell something was wrong and finally coaxed the story out of her. This was when I was struck by the realization of how much she needed me to be with her. She was still in the fight, but she had been hit hard.

During this time I was blessed to see her start to come back; she had been very distant, unable to hold a conversation, and it was with much difficulty that she was able to communicate her needs and wants. Fortunately, we were close enough that in most cases, even though the words would not come, I would get the idea, and could help her express herself. I shared with my boss the difficulty that travel was causing, and he graciously told me that unless it was just vital that I could work from home, the decision on where to work had been the right one. We tried letting her stay with her parents when I would have to travel, and they did their best to take care of her, but they both have health issues of their own, and Barbie, being Barbie even in the midst of all, would try to assume the role of care giver when she was with them, this would cause her to get tired and many times lead to falls, and it was very hard for them to help her up. Many family members offered to help or stay with her, but to me while the willingness was there in most cases the ability wasn't. Most of our family was aging and did not have the strength to help her up without hurting her. And maybe I was the one who had the problem, but my girl needed me there. This stage of our life lasted about eight months. We did not go many places because we wanted to stay away from people, as her immunity was down from time to time. She spent two or three weeks in the hospital from an infection. She also had a hiatal hernia and acid reflux, and the solution was more pills.

During this time, she was weak a lot and experienced a lot of fatigue. We went for a long period that we could not get to church. Still, our faith had been and continued to be the bedrock foundation in our lives. We could smile and laugh in the face of this trial because of Jesus living in our hearts, and His grace, and His peace.

6 Be careful for nothing; but in every thing by prayer and supplication with thanksgiving let your requests be made known unto God.

7 And the peace of God, which passeth all understanding, shall keep your hearts and minds through Christ Jesus. (Php 4:6-7)

This peace keeps us going, so since we were separated from our church, we decided to have our own. During this time of study, and many hours of heart-to-heart talks, scripture reading, and meditation on what we had read, we experienced some liberating growth. I became more accepting of God's will in our lives, believing that He knows what is best and believing His promises. I tried diligently to make sure Barbie was along on this, but found out later while reading her journals she was way ahead of me. Some of the things that occurred to me at this time were:

• We do not die because we are well or sick, young or old, we die because we are alive. Once life begins, once we are born, there is an appointment that all will meet.

Heb 9:27 And as it is appointed unto men once to die, but after this the judgment:
• We all have that appointment set, we can hasten it, but it will not be put off. Maybe He knows something coming in our life that we don't.

Isa 57:1 The righteous perisheth, and no man layeth it to heart: and merciful men are taken away, none considering that the righteous is taken away from the evil to come.
2 He shall enter into peace: they shall rest in their beds, each one walking in his uprightness.

These and many other things were made clear to me. Now, you may be thinking that I did not get down, or see the darkness, or question God. Well, I did. Some will tell you that you should not question God, but I disagree. If you have questions, ask. If you are mad at Him, tell Him. I did all of these things. He already knows our heart, so we will not surprise Him, but we may surprise ourselves. It is through these times of pouring our heart out about the good and the bad, the best and the worst, that we can heal. I got answers to my questions, and maybe a rebuke or two for my anger, but I did not carry it around. I realized that life and death go hand and hand, just like Barbie and I. We all have that appointment coming, and we cannot avoid it. As far as the separation here, it will be no easier when we are ninety then it would be today. What we were experiencing is life, and we again were experiencing a very dark time. But as one of my favorite passages on the Bible, a passage that is found throughout states: *And it came to pass*

There is a blessing in knowing that when troubles come. They do not come to stay, but as with everything, they will pass.

She continued to do her therapy, worked out at home, completed her chemo, and as always fought. When I asked her after one of our early doctor appointments what she was going to do, she said, "I am going to fight; if I don't fight, I will die." And that is what she did. Her MRI after eight months revealed no appreciable tumor, and again the fight to normal begins. She was left this time with what seemed to be permanent weakness to her right side, and the inability to think about things before she acts, which makes her staying by herself still not an option, but we did return to our regular church schedule, our Friday night date night, and for the most part, our wonderful blessed life. She continued with dogged determination to get back to her normal life; we anxiously wait to see if that is God's will for our lives or not, but whatever His will is for our life, we know it is the best for us.

Chapter 12
The Girl in the Fight
and the Fight in the Girl

After the last MRI that revealed all clear, we again worked our way back to a normal life. Barbie exercised her arm and leg and fought to keep all of her mobility; it was a very hard eight months of chemo that had left her fatigued and weak. One thing that struck me and speaks volumes about who she is, was in reading the stack of her journals beginning from about a year after the last surgery until just before that Sunday morning, I have found no entries where she feels sorry for herself or even writing about her tumor or anything it has cost her. I find her writing about the normal things of life that affect everyone – needing to diet, issues with our son, maybe with her husband (not sure, may need to read again), often about people she has met and their problems, writing short prayers for them – but she had never let this steal her goal of having a normal life. She had never been the girl fighting cancer; she was just Barbie. I intended to add journal entries to show how she felt about her fight and its effects on her, but instead I will try to put some entries showing the lack of effect on her and of a fight won.

The entries below refer to her cousin, who was diagnosed in 2007 with a glioblastoma. I did not know how she would react to this considering her experience, but she reacted like Barbie:

> *10/20/2007*
>
> *I stopped and got Kevin and his Son two hot dogs, we stopped and visited Kevin, he is getting worse, walking with a cane and walker, I did his dishes, his son came back, I told him that I got him a hot dog also, he ate it and he started cooking sausage links. I took over and made them gravy and biscuits, fixed Kevin's plate and we left, I feel sad for Kevin, maybe worse for his son. I feel good that I stopped by to see him; I'll stop by next week also.*

She continued to visit and help in any way possible, as long as he stayed at home, and was a regular visitor after he went into the nursing home.

> *12/20/2007*
>
> *We got ready went outside, Dave started the car, Grandpa came and we left, got there, Kevin was asleep in an awkward position, twisted and turning, his head going one way, his body another. I went to see Elsie, and a lady was pushing her in a wheelchair, I followed them to her lunch room, they were waiting for their lunch, but it was 1 pm, I talked for a while. I went to see Kevin, he was awake, but out of his mind, we spoke for a while, he went back to sleep, we left.*

Kevin passed away a couple of months after that entry.

This one is a reoccurring theme through all of the years of her journals:

10/01/06
I went back into the Church welcoming people and my Mom and Dad walked in the doors, I was told that Geneva called them up and asked if they would come! It was a glorious moment in my life, to see them come. I was so happy; I started crying tears of joy! I was so proud; I told the whole Church that my Mom and Dad came, thank you Lord.

12/30/07
The Lord wants all of the unsaved people, regardless of their sins! I was there, everyone was there, I hope my Mom & Dad get that feeling in their hearts, God's love is unconditional, forever, I want my parents to feel that kind of love from God, in their hearts & Souls forever, I hope one day if you wish Lord.

2Pe 3:9 The Lord is not slack concerning his promise, as some men count slackness; but is longsuffering to us-ward, not willing that any should perish, but that all should come to repentance.

Jesus died for all, and God calls all to repentance, the choice is always ours and it will be made, not choosing, is choosing.

Her concern for the neighbors who were sick, especially

when there was a terminal prognosis never ceases to amaze me. I think she saw it as her duty to come along beside those folks to be an inspiration to them; she feels that is part of why she went through her trials, to help others who go through the same. To me, it seemed only right after the community had done the same for us, we always agreed to also help out monetarily, as much as we could, and Barbie was always quick to want to go see those who are suffering, to give them a hug, and to comfort anyway she could. That is what was done for us. Words are hard to find to express how much it helped. Someone to talk to, sometimes about what you are going through, and sometimes about anything other than that, or a little extra money, can relieve the pressure for just a little while, and every little bit helps.

A neighbor just up the road was also diagnosed with a Glioblastoma, and it progressed very rapidly, as it is prone to do. Barbie wanted to visit him often, and he was always very happy to see her, at first in his home talking about what they both had been through, then in the hospital. Even when the ability to talk had left him, he made clear that he was glad to see her. She continued to visit as long as he knew her and did all she could to comfort his family after he departed. This is typical of who she is; she very seldom buys or wants anything for herself, she loves to shop and spend on other people. I have found that it is not uncommon to see her crying about someone else's hardships either in our day to day life or someone she sees on television. Just recently upon starting her new chemo, hair loss can be a problem, and since that day years ago when she cried as I cut it, she has regrown her long beautiful hair. This time as we cut it, to again try to mitigate her loss, there were no tears, and she packaged up the fourteen-inch ponytail and sent it off for wigs to be made for cancer patients. To this day, if we are in church or around people and someone is crying, she has to get up and make her way over to them – even in the times when it was questionable if she could make it without falling – give them a hug, and cry with them if needed.

> *June 12, 2008*
> *I slept in the front room (someone snoring), turned on the news and saw that the Boy Scout group had been hit by a tornado, four dead, you never know what could happen to anyone, enjoy life.*

This is a lasting thought she has gotten from her trail, we found out that life can change in an instant, we need to take joy where and when we find it, because it can become elusive very quickly.

> *June 20 2008*
> *We went to the bank in Chesapeake, Dave went in, I stayed in the car, I saw a young girl sitting in a truck, she smiled at me and I smiled back, the Mother got in the truck, when she got in she smacked her face so hard, and called her trash. The girl said I did not say anything and of course she was crying, her mother told her to keep her mouth shut or she would get another slap. I told Dave what her mother said, it made me mad and sad because I was there a long time ago.*

We talked often in the earlier days about her conflict with

her mom when she was younger, and how it left her with hard feelings. Then after she was saved, she slowly started to forgive. It took her a while; long open wounds heal hard, but she knew that since she had been forgiven that she needed to forgive. When she finally did, she found out what everyone does who can find it in their heart to forgive – the one doing the forgiving is the one that is released. Her anger or our anger that we carry around does not affect the one it is directed to. They might not even know we are angry with them; it only affects the one carrying it. A wondrous thing happened – that anger was replaced with a deep love and care for her parents that we read about in her journals.

Around this time, her best friend Sam passed away. She had lung cancer and went very slowly and painfully. We spent quite a bit of time in hospice sitting and talking with her when she could, just sitting when she could not. Sam had been a good friend to Barbie for many years; they had always been close. with deep appreciation I recall that Sam encouraged Barbie to date me (and I thought it was my idea!); I owe you one, Sam. It seemed that we were spending a lot of time in hospitals, homes of the sick and funerals, the words dad spoke many years before came to me often, about how many people were feeling sorry for Barbie whose appointment was coming before hers, and they had no idea it was coming. We need to make sure we are ready, because our name may be called at any time.

2Co 6:1 We then, as workers together with him, beseech you also that ye receive not the grace of God in vain.

2 (For he saith, I have heard thee in a time accepted, and in the day of salvation have I succoured thee: behold, now is the accepted time; behold, now is the day of salvation.)

Today is the only day we know that we have. Tomorrow may not come.

> *June 8, 2008*
> *Dave took me to Wilson Cemetery, Kevin has a tombstone, and it's very pretty, I gave flowers to Grandma, Stacy, Kevin and Sam, Dave said Sam will be dead four years in November; it does not seem that long ago. It does not seem that long, I still think about her and Doug often, of the good times we had, my friends and family seem to go so fast, I better enjoy.*

We learned that going through trials like this will do a couple of things in your life. First, it rearranges your priorities and makes clear what is important in life. The things most people spend time and energy worrying and arguing about do not amount to much when compared to life and death, and only facing death will make that clear. You learn real quick who your friends are, and more importantly who they are not; the results of this are surprising. And when tested you learn (or maybe those around you learn) if you have faith or not, this is why Barbie can worry about others and not herself, she knows her future and is steadfast in her faith, she does not need to be worried about.

Joh 14:1 Let not your heart be troubled: ye believe in God, believe also in me.

2 In my Father's house are many mansions: if it were not so, I would have told you. I go to prepare a place for you.

3 And if I go and prepare a place for you, I will come again, and receive you unto myself; that where I am, there ye may be also.

4 And whither I go ye know, and the way ye know.

5 Thomas saith unto him, Lord, we know not whither thou goest; and how can we know the way?

6 Jesus saith unto him, I am the way, the truth, and the life: no man cometh unto the Father, but by me.

This is where Barbie's peace comes from. She knows that she has a home and that Jesus will come and take her there when the time comes.

Much of her journaling involved recording the church service and notes on the message; apparently this is how she learned and retained, by writing it down. Her life is about her lord, her church, her son, her husband (a truly lucky man), her family, and her community. She has a very hard time expressing this anymore, but those of us that are lucky enough to know her and to know her heart still know it. She has always very much enjoyed life and can find joy in the little things, like her birthday, which is celebrated every year for one week. She relishes each new year and is thankful for it. She also loves Christmas; when she can, she puts up her Christmas village, tree and various decorations around the house and truly enjoys the season. This ability to find joy in the small things has never changed; you can see her smile as she watches the birds at her feeder or the calves running in the field or any baby, animal or human in life or on television. If we are in a restaurant, and a family with a baby sits close, I dine alone; she is still sitting there, but only in body, I have figured out in watching, this may just be part of being a woman. We can go into a doctor office for any kind of treatment, and there have been many different ones, and almost with our fail, I will hear, "Did you see that poor person, I feel so sorry for them." I have heard this at times when I was holding on to her arm so she would not fall, and still Her problems are not what she sees.

So in my attempt to relay how sorry she has felt for herself and how she sat around and wondered "Why me?" the volumes written about her regrets, I failed. Instead, what I got was a wonderful blessing of reading about the normal life we have enjoyed, the fight she has put up for years with fatigue, a fight not shared with anyone. She worked to do what every wife and mother did, and took any extra weight she had to carry in stride. I read of a wife deeply in love with her very lucky husband who missed him when he was gone and looked forward eagerly to his return, and loving to travel along anytime the opportunity was made available. I read of a blessed life that I am truly grateful to be a part of.

The reading of her journals has been a great blessing to me. Many years have past since she has been able to carry on a long conversation, to express what is in her heart, to have those long heart-to-heart talks. The reading of these thoughts recorded over the years is like being let back into a place that I miss very much. It has been like sitting down and having a long conversation, ones like we used to have daily. As I sit and type this and feel the tears roll down my cheeks, I realize just how much I miss her lost abilities.

We got about a year reprieve from the chemo, then came the routine visit after she had completed her second three-month MRI. We again watched as the doctor walked in, the expression on the face giving away the gravity of the news he was about to deliver, and again we got the news we did not want to hear, "Your tumor is growing again." Again the discussion of treatment options was before us. This time Barbie listened intently to the options and settled on the decision with the demeanor of a fighter who has participated in many bouts, her experience showing.

Chapter 13
The Privilege of Caregiving

I have often been thankful to have been counted worthy by both our Lord and Barbie to be trusted with her care when she is in need. There is no way to state the awesome privilege to be trusted by someone you love to the extent that their well-being would be placed into your hands.

I had never given any thought to being placed into this situation when I was younger. We were young, healthy and at that time in very good physical condition. The idea that I may have to take care of Barbie had never even crossed my mind briefly. We worked from daylight to dark side by side, and I was often pressed to keep up. When the time came, I did not really even consider it or give any thought to the implications or the responsibilities. She had a need, and I was the only choice to meet that need. I was not going to trust anyone else. Now I just needed to develop the skills that I needed to do the job. I have been fortunate to have grown up in an environment where I saw both parents cooking or doing any task needed. My dad is a very good cook, doing mostly the traditional home cooking, so it was not a stretch that I learned to cook early. One of my memories of learning to cook came with my sister-in-law, who is a couple of years older that me. We were staying at our house one day while mom and dad worked outside at something. We decided that we wanted to make sausage gravy. She had not made it before, and neither had I, but I had seen it done on several occasions, so we made a valiant attempt. The result was a thick paste-like substance that could easily have been sliced to make sandwiches, but it did taste surprisingly like sausage gravy. Our next attempt was much better. Over the years, I had become quite proficient at several dishes in addition to the staples. So it was not a big stretch when I took over the cooking and cleaning for the family. I was surprised at the feeling of satisfaction that I experienced at being able to take on her task. The love I felt for her not only drove me to take on her task but to want to do them well.

What was totally foreign to me was the medical aspect, changing bandages, dressing and cleaning wounds, watching for side effects, and a host of other terrifying task that came with the job. But if that was what she needed, than that is what I would learn to do. At the time, she did not have the ability to know what needed to be done or to take care of it, so I eagerly looked for and to the best of my abilities provided for all of her needs.

There were many offers of help, and I appreciated them all, but many of the tasks to be performed were very personal, and I did not want to subject Barbie to any embarrassment by having other people helping her with personal issues. She quickly began to look to me for her needs and care. Looking back, one thing that I may have done wrong was I tend to do too much for her. I hate to see her struggle with things, and instead of letting her, I did things for her, and I have discovered that it may be better for her to struggle through things on the way back to doing them for herself. It is a habit that I have discovered after you start is very hard to break. I have mentioned her looking to me for words when she is struggling to find them; I find that I have a hard time letting her try to get them, and maybe improve, when I know what she is trying to say, and I can relieve her struggle by telling her. The harder her life became, the easier I wanted to try to make it. I wrote earlier about not having regrets, and I do not want to be left thinking that I should have done more for her when she needed me to.

Mt 19:5 And said, For this cause shall a man leave father and mother, and shall cleave to his wife: and they twain shall be one flesh?

6 Wherefore they are no more twain, but one flesh. What therefore God hath joined together, let not man put asunder.

When we took our vows, I took each one to heart, I was always raised to be a man of my word, if I do not mean it, then do not say it. Barbie and I have talked and laughed. We have literally been in every situation that we vowed. We have been poorer, although we have never been destitute, we defiantly qualified as poorer, we have been richer, again never rich but better than when we were poorer. We have seen the better, as well as the worse, we have enjoyed perfect health and everything that comes with that, and we have seen the sickness. And through it all we have loved and cherished each other. Now how can one enjoy and endure all the good that is brought into your life, and not stand with your spouse through the bad when it comes? I never have liked hearing a wedding where the couple have written their own vows and replaced the traditional; I feel it is very important to take those vows and to consider them, because there is a good chance that these will be what are to be faced in this life. In taking these vows, when in sickness we have not only the duty but the honor of acting as the caregiver for our spouse, we are the one that is to be counted on. Think about what an expression of love it is to trust someone with your very life and well-being, and what an honor it is to be that person who is trusted.

Lu: 12; 48 For unto whomsoever much is given, of him shall be much required: and to whom men have committed much, of him they will ask the more.

When we are married our spouse committed much to us, we will be ask more, only life as it plays out will reveal the extent, but remember much has been given. When I think of the things that I have been given, I am humbled, I have the love of a wonderful woman, one who is in my corner and stands behind me regardless of the opposition, a best friend who will never forsake me, and I know that the one thing that I can count in is Barbie backing me up. Our pastor will kid with her, he will get on me a little, and it is just a second before she is calling him down. I have been given a constant companion someone who will always be there to help me to the best of her abilities.

Ge 2:18 And the LORD God said, It is not good that the man should be alone; I will make him an help meet for him.

I have a partner in every venture, someone who is pulling for me to succeed at anything I do. I smile when I come in from hunting or fishing, as the very first thing I hear is, 'Did you get one?" If I say no she says, "well shoot." If I have been successful, she is as happy if not happier that I am. Yes, much has been given me and I count it an honor to be there in her time of need. I just hope that I can be looked upon by her as one who can be counted on as she is, as the one in her corner and standing beside her. I hope – no I pray – that the Lord always will give me the grace to never let her down when she needs me. I know beyond the shadow of a doubt that if I was the one who was sick and in the need of help that she would be there, attending to my every need, doing all the things for me that I could not do, if the shoe was on the other foot, I would have the best caregiver that could be had, and it is my great privilege to try to be that for her.

There are great rewards for being there for someone you love in their time of need, as I have mentioned, we have drawn closer than we could have ever imagined, I get to spend more time with the one who I love the most in this world, and I know that I am needed and appreciated. Just to see the look of love in her eyes is reward enough for a life time. There is also great pain any time the one you love is hurting or sick yet you cannot do anything to help. You feel the pain of helplessness, and even though you are a great help you wish you could do more.

I think God for trusting me to help one of His children when she is in need. It has not all been easy, there have been nights when she has passed out, fell and hurt herself, had seizures, burnt herself, had pneumonia, UTIs, trips to the emergency room in the middle of the night, and all of these coming with their own special care needs, but much like I learned crop insurance, I have learned nursing the same way. I have become quite proficient at diagnosing problems, bandaging wounds, changing dressings, and doing all the things that once scared me. I also have gained many other skills that I would have never anticipated needing, things like hairdressing, I have been the only one to cut Barbie's hair since that day, when she was standing in the bathroom crying as I cut it. The good thing is she does not cry anymore, as I have learned to apply makeup and curl hair. However, I have not mastered painting fingernails; it seems to take a steadier hand than I possess. All of these things I count as a joy to be able to do for her, when I can see her look in the mirror and smile I am paid in full, although I do not always get that smile because I said I learned to do all those things, that does not mean I do them all well. You never know just what you can do until you are put into a position where things need to be done, and you are the one who needs to do them, there is a great since of pleasure from being able to provide for a need that is encountered by someone you love. There are times when we all go through things that seem to be too hard, or the burden seems to get too heavy, but others have gone through what we are going through and they made it, so always remember we can too.

1Co 10:12 Wherefore let him that thinketh he standeth take heed lest he fall.

13 There hath no temptation taken you but such as is common to man: but God is faithful, who will not suffer you to be tempted above that ye are able; but will with the temptation also make a way to escape, that ye may be able to bear it.

We have the ability and the power to deal with what we are faced with. We only have to tap into the truth and his power. We need to always remember there is a plan, and its ending is good, I have expressed many times the blessings and the joy we have both derived from our storm, and I am sure there is more to come.

For I know the thoughts that I think toward you, saith the LORD, thoughts of peace, and not of evil, to give you an expected end. (Jer 29:11)

He knows the end from the beginning, and he has promised good to those who love him, but that does not mean that the path may not be rough, so we just walk and take joy where we can find it, always drawing on the peace that passeth all understanding. Many times I feel that peace and just marvel at how it can be present at this time in my life, but I guess that if I understood it, then I would not have the peace that passeth all understanding.

So I encourage you, if you find yourself thrust into the terrifying position of needing to be a caregiver to someone in need, throw yourself into the job wholeheartedly. The rewards will be greater than you ever imagined. It will be hard at times, it will probably be scary at times, you will make mistakes and learn from them, but we do what we have to do for those we love. When your loved one looks at you with the look that shows you that they are not worried because they know you are there for them, and their eyes are filled with love, it is worth every effort that you have put forth.

I will give you a piece of profound advice that may help you out: If you are going to have to learn to cook and you are starting from scratch, get a dog. They will eat anything.

Chapter 14
Present Time, the Fight Goes On
She Would Not Change the Past if She Could

Again we find ourselves sitting in a doctor's office, looking at an MRI and seeing the tumor that is being pointed out. This time is a little different, the shock is gone, and we realize this is the fight before us and Barbie is in it. We discuss treatment options; and as a group decided that she should see the radiation doctor to see if there are any new options since the last time we visited. We left the appointment disappointed but accepting of the fact that her fight was not over. As we rode home, we reminisced of just how good of a life we enjoy, and how that her disease was a big part of what had made our life what it is. As we got home, I asked her if she had her fight on. She said, "Tomorrow." I said, "Good enough." Sometimes you just need to be sad a little while. We talked and she was a little down, no crying, no lamenting her situation, just a girl taking a break from the fight. We got ready later and went to church, we told all of our loved ones there of the doctor's appointment, and the news we had received, and ask for an interest in their prayers. There were many tears when we talked to my mother, and again when we talked to hers. It seemed a little strange that those who loved us were taking it harder than she was. As I talked to her mother, who by the way never had come to church or Jesus, it was apparent that she was taking it very hard. I told her that she was grieving as those who had no hope, and that is not how we were going to handle this.

1Th 4:13 But I would not have you to be ignorant, brethren, concerning them which are asleep, that ye sorrow not, even as others which have no hope.

Not only do we have hope, we posses it. It is not at all like man who hopes something good will happen; our hope is a possession that we will redeem when the time comes.

The day came, and we visited our radiologist. As we talked, he told us that there had been advances since the last time we were there, and he thought that a on-time radiation treatment may take care of the tumor. Over the next few days, he studied the MRI and her past records and determined that the area that needed to be treated was not in the area that had been treated before, a good thing since that area has received the maximum lifetime dose of radiation. He told us that it was close, though, and he thought it would be better to break the single dose into five, administered at a rate of two per week. He gave us a minute, and we discussed, and as with the previous decision, much to my relief, she was the one making it. My mind in these times often go back to that very first occurrence, which at this time is approaching 17 years ago, to the life and death decision that I had to make for her, absolutely the hardest thing I have ever done in my life. Thanks be unto God, it seems to have been the right one. She decided that she would go with the focused radiation. The appointment was made to begin later that week.

The day came, and I helped her into the office. The new occurrence had left her very weak and unstable again, unable to walk on her own without falling. She took the first treatment in stride, came out a little spacy and confused, but that passed quickly. She was left fatigued and rested a lot the next couple of days. The next four treatments went much the same – they left her very tired and fatigued, but she slowly got her strength back. Very soon after the last treatment, she was talking and getting words better, and I was overjoyed to see that her balance was getting better, but she would have to battle though the fatigue, a battle that would stretch out over several months, before we would know how her mobility would be. We talked often about her fight, and she assured me she was in it. She worked some on her stationary bike but was left with very little endurance. Grocery shopping involved more walking than she could stand, but she was getting stronger little by little.

Her three-month MRI came and went with no surprises, and she continued to get stronger, the seventeen year anniversary of her first surgery came and went and it appeared that maybe we were back on the right road. She worked much harder than most realize to live her life, and I try to never forget to tell her how proud of her that I am. I have never met anyone like her. Many would have given up, but the darker things get the more it strengthens her resolve. From listening to stories from her past, this may be the same trait that made her adolescence so rough, the inability to back down that cost her in her youth serves her very well now. She continued through the next months getting stronger, her speech getting better, and before long she was in better condition that she had been in the last two or three years, it seemed that normal was only a few months away. Many probably had not realized how far from normal life had been during that time, she had fell a lot, I had to be within sight of her most of the time to be able to help her around, if I was not she would try on her own. This has led to a very in active lifestyle for me, not what I was used to, but that was OK, it is our fight, and with the Lord's help, we are up to it.

The six-month MRI rolled around, and we went into it confident that it would show what we were seeing every day. The follow-up visit came, and as the doctor walked in, we could see by his face that it was going to be another one of those visits. He shared with us that the tumor was growing yet again, and in the three months since her last scan it had reached a size of eight mm. after discussing the options we decided the Doctor would discuss her case with the tumor board that was convening the following week. After that meeting, it was decided that another type of MRI should be performed, this one should differentiate between radiation necrosis and tumor, it was suspected that since it was in the same area, it could be residual effect from the radiation. When the results came back, they confirmed it as tumor growth, so the treatment discussion of radiation was out since it was the same area, leaving her with only the two chemo treatment options. It was decided that since the one she had been on was fairly well-tolerated and had been effective that she would resume the same treatment. Blood test were performed medication was ordered and insurance was dealt with, and all the time she continues to improve. We again have the talks that we have had many times, the positive change that has taken place in our lives, the fact that we can now actually thank God for it, and understand that the good things that happen in our lives, do not look good all of the time. We were getting closer to the place the apostle Paul spoke of:

Php 4:11 Not that I speak in respect of want: for I have learned, in whatsoever state I am, therewith to be content.

12 I know both how to be abased, and I know how to abound: every where and in all things I am instructed both to be full and to be hungry, both to abound and to suffer need.

13 I can do all things through Christ which strengtheneth me.

This is a lesson that I think can only be learned through great trails, when you realize that you cannot let your joy be a direct result of your situation, and then you can move to this place. We decided a long time ago that we would not let cancer steal our joy, each day when we awake we have been given another day together, we can choose if we want to take pleasure in it, or let it be taken from us, we will take the pleasure of each day that we can.

I had been talking with our pastor and confiding in him that I was going to need to try to find someone to stay with Barbie sometimes when I traveled, it was hard for her to stay in the motel by herself, and I had been with my new company about a year now and needed to step up my performance. No one was saying anything, and as a matter of fact when I had talked to the president of the company and expressed that to him, his response was "You are right where you need to be." I agreed, but felt I needed to be doing more, again this has re-affirmed the fact that I had been led to the right decision when taking my job.

Our pastor said we would pray about it, and maybe the

Lord would put someone in our lives that we needed. Within two or three weeks a young lady who was married to a wonderful young brother at church came forward and was saved, we had visited and talked before, and her love for Barbie was obvious. I talked it over with Barbie and we decided to approach her about taking the job of staying with Barbie as I traveled, she was out of work, and being newly saved she needed to be away from bad influences in her life, as we talked it was apparent that we both needed this. We talked and an agreement was reached, she would help out one day a week and stay overnight or through the day as needed. She was a perfect fit; she had some home health training, and had come out of a hard family situation where she had to deal with parents having seizures, so she was not intimidated by the prospects of what could come. We had a long talk about many scary things that could possible come to pass, the possibility of falls, seizures, emergency room visits, calmly she took notes and gathered information she felt would be needed if these things were to happen in my absence. She and Barbie get along wonderfully and when I have to leave I am confident that Barbie is in good hands, another prayer answered, and in a way that left no doubt of the source of the answer, it is a wonderful thing when you know your prayers are heard.

She completed two thirty day cycles of her meds and went back for a follow up MRI to see what was going on, we again went in confident that all was going well, after all, she seemed to continue to improve, and again the doctors face contradicted. He explained to us that the tumor had increased to thirteen mm while taking the chemo, the doctor look on with a puzzled look on his face as Barbie did not react to the news, she simply ask "What are my options?" The doctor explained that Barbie could continue on the current medicine or try the other. He told us of the possible side effects, which were many. The cycle would start with a dose of pills, followed in eight days by an infusion of a different drug, and then a third drug would be started, more pills that would be taken for two weeks. Without hesitation, Barbie said that's the one I will take. You could see his surprise to her decision made without emotion:

(Heb 10:9) Having therefore, brethren, boldness to enter into the holiest by the blood of Jesus,

20 By a new and living way, which he hath consecrated for us, through the veil, that is to say, his flesh;

21 And having an high priest over the house of God;

22 Let us draw near with a true heart in full assurance of faith, having our hearts sprinkled from an evil conscience, and our bodies washed with pure water.

23 Let us hold fast the profession of our faith without wavering; (for he is faithful that promised;)

24 And let us consider one another to provoke unto love and to good works

What Barbie's young doctor did not understand is that she could and regularly did boldly approach the throne of God with her prayers and she had learned not to waiver. This is a difficult lesson learned in hardships.

Barbie shared her thoughts with me on her decision. The drug she was on was not working, so the decisions was an easy one, try the other one. Again meds were ordered, and a port had to be inserted, she had this done and went through the healing period, one evening as we set at dinner, talking after we had finished, the conversation again turned to our lives and the past, I asked her that if she could go back and change anything, would she? I assumed that anyone who had went through what she had, even though she has great faith and trust God for her future, surely she would say, "I would go back and not have my tumor," but this time I was the one taken off guard. She simply looked at me and said no I would not. As we talked about it, we discussed the path that we had walked, the fact that we had come out of a lifestyle that was not very good, and into one that involved church, honesty, and much cleaner living, and how that if that change had not taken place, how either of us may not be alive now, and how we would never know, but maybe her six month prognosis could have lengthened either one of our lives if not both, how that because of her disease. When I returned to work, I insisted on a position with benefits, that led to better pay, steady work and security and how without that, maybe we would have fell, as many couple do to arguments over money or the lack of it, and possibly split up because of that. How that even though it had been rough time for us and I am sure for him, that now our son is in a good place, and how that even a small change could have set us on a different course, she said no, I would not change a thing.

The Lord has truly supplied the Grace to us as we have needed it. We have had time of doubt, times of weakness, times of anger, which ultimately have resulted in times of growth, he has proved himself faithful time and time again, and is true in all things, he has proven this to me.

(2Co 12:9) And he said unto me, My grace is sufficient for thee: for my strength is made perfect in weakness. Most gladly therefore will I rather glory in my infirmities, that the power of Christ may rest upon me.

10 Therefore I take pleasure in infirmities, in reproaches, in necessities, in persecutions, in distresses for Christ's sake: for when I am weak, then am I strong.

I have found that we do not discover our strength until we discover our weakness, when we get to the end of our ability and realize that we are lacking, and everything is spiraling out of control and there is nothing we can do about it, and then is when we can hear him call.

As I finish our story, Barbie has just started her new treatment. We visited our radiologist this week and he looked at her last MRI, he said he had to wonder if it is actually tumor, or if it may be necrosis, but that he would not contradict the radiologist who had read the scans. This was a ray of hope as he was the same doctor who said her original tumor was not returning before her third surgery which produced only scar tissue. The plan now is to take the treatment and see how the spot reacts, no reaction would indicate necrosis, any reaction would confirm tumor. Barbie still has her fight on and had not effects from the first dose of meds, she continues to enjoy life and we are pledged to do so as long as we have it.

Some may question why did we not wait until the treatment was complete and share the outcome. This book was never intended to be about the outcome. The book is to be about hope, when we first took the plunge into darkness, I sought out survivor stories, I looked for any hope to lay hold on, and it can be hard to come by. We want to give this to those who have taken that plunge and who desperately need to find some hope to grab on to, I encourage you to take Barbie's story as hope, and that you look to the one true hope Jesus, without whom this would have been a most bleak story. As I have said before, death does not come from sickness or health, it comes from life, it is as much a part of life as breath, so while we have breath we need to prepare for that appointment that we all have in our future.

(Ro 10:9) That if thou shalt confess with thy mouth the Lord Jesus, and shalt believe in thine heart that God hath raised him from the dead, thou shalt be saved.

10 For with the heart man believeth unto righteousness; and with the mouth confession is made unto salvation.

11 For the scripture saith, Whosoever believeth on him shall not be ashamed.

This is the greatest help that I could give anyone who is going through tough times, or who is not, because in this life one thing is for sure, we will not get out without having troubles, if you have not had any yet, be thankful and get ready. The one true constant through our trial has been his grace, which has given us the ability to face each part of our trial, and it is the one sure thing in our future, we will continue to enjoy each day we have together and look to his grace when the end comes, because sick or not it will come, and his grace will be sufficient, I will end with the words from a wonderful song called "New Grace":

All of grace is my story
All the way from Earth to Glory
Since by grace He lifted me from sin and woe
Living grace He has extended
As on Him my heart depended
He'll give new grace when it's my time to go.
Grace not yet discovered
Grace not yet uncovered
Grace from His bountiful store
Grace to cross the river
And grace to face forever

But there'll be new grace I've not needed before.
There's been grace for every mile
There's been grace for every trial
There's been grace sufficient from His vast supply
Grace to make my heart more tender
Grace to love and pray for sinners
But there'll be new grace when it's my time to die.
Grace not yet discovered
Grace not yet uncovered
Grace from His bountiful store
Grace to cross the river
And grace to face forever
But there'll be new grace I've not needed before.

Chapter 15
Answered Prayers, Listening to His Voice

One of the oldest enduring questions ask is, why do bad things happen to good people, probably a better or just as relevant question would be; why good things happen to any of us. We often question the bad but take the good in stride, as it is what should happen to us. One of the greatest lessons that I have learned is to look back at blessings and answered prayers in our life.

Job 2:9 Then said his wife unto him, Dost thou still retain thine integrity? curse God, and die.

10 But he said unto her, Thou speakest as one of the foolish women speaketh. What? shall we receive good at the hand of God, and shall we not receive evil? In all this did not Job sin with his lips.

If we have accepted the good in our life with or without thanksgiving, how can we not also accept the bad? In this life we are not promised that we will not have problems, actually it is just the opposite. Problems are just a part of life, if we are fortunate we may go a long time without them, if so be thankful.

I think of all the prayers that were said for Barbie, as we have went through the years, prayers from family, brothers and sisters from the area churches, from coworkers and a multitude of strangers who have heard of our battle by word of mouth. We are very grateful for each prayer that has been said on our account and do not discount the effect that they have had. We have no doubt that they have been heard and attended to, but also just knowing that someone cares enough to stop their day, their life, and spend some time interceding for you, it helps.

I think of the times that we have seen prayers answered in our lives, the times that God has spoken to us. I have talked about the times that Barbie has heard his voice, the times the still small voice from within has spoken to me. But looking back we can see his voice in many ways. There was the time that our son was having emergency surgery to remove his spleen. I was working out of town when Barbie received the call that he has collapsed in the gym at school. Barbie rushed to his side as the emergency squad picked him up and took him to the hospital. She called me from the hospital, and I started the long trip home from northern Ohio. I made it and found them in a hospital room, test had been performed and a ruptured spleen was the diagnosis. It would have to be removed the next morning. We spent a long night in the hospital watching in helplessness, as he lay in pain. The next morning we and the family were gathered in the waiting room, and many prayers had been said. Barbie was a nervous wreck as is to be expected; as the day wore on, she tried to keep it together. As we sat in the waiting room she for some reason put her hand in between the chair arm and the seat, feeling something she drew it out. When we looked she was holding a small angel that had been a part of a neckless, what had been a neckless to someone else, was God speaking comfort to a worried mother now. He speaks to us many times, but often we are just not listening. Many times I have poured out my heart in prayer, then after a few minutes opened the Bible and started to read. Many times I would open to what seemed to be a random scripture, only to find that it spoke to exactly what I had been praying about. Or upon attending the next church service the preacher would preach a message that sounded as if he had been listening to my prayers.

There are other times when He speaks much louder. My dad was up on the hill cutting hay; I had been on the road working and had just made my way home. For some reason, dad had taken his truck up on the hill that day and parked it, something that he did not usually do. On this day, it would prove to be a life saver. As he worked, there was a problem with the mowing machine. The tractor had a bad starter, so he parked it on a bank to work on the mowing machine. When he finished he climbed on the tractor and pushed the clutch in so it would start to roll, he would then let out the clutch and start the tractor. This time when he got on the tractor and pushed the clutch it did not roll. At this time, dad was in his early seventies, he got off of the tractor and pushed on the back tire until it started to roll, then he went around the tire and stepped up on the step located in front of the back tire. The back tire of the tractor was loaded with calcium for extra weight, each tire weighed about a thousand pounds plus the weight of the tractor. As he stepped on with one foot, the back tire caught the other, pulling him off and landing him in front of the tire as the tractor picked up speed. The tractor ran over him, starting at the hip, and going diagonally over his chest and off his shoulder. After lying for a minute, he got up out of the field and made his way to the truck. He started off of the hill and lost his vision. Knowing he was in trouble, he attempted to drive by memory to get out to the gravel road which lay about a mile away. As the drove the truck veered into the hay field, and he drove along side of a ditch drawing nearer and nearer to a wood line. Feeling that he was no longer on the road, dad stopped and said this prayer. "Lord if I am going to live through this, I am going to need your help" He tells that almost immediately after finishing this prayer, his eyesight returned. Seeing that he was about to drive into the woods, he turned the truck and got back on the driveway and drove to my house. I had been home about fifteen minutes when he pulled into the driveway laying on the horn. We called 911 and let them know I was bringing him to the ambulance station, and he was rushed to the hospital. He had broken all the ribs on one side of his body and cracked all of the ribs on the other side; he also had a broken wrist. He made a full recovery. Later my brother and I walked the path he had drove while blinded by pain, thinking about neighbors who had been killed by tractor accidents, we heard the Lord again that day on that walk. There was no doubt that he had answered dad's prayer.

1Ki 19:11 And he said, Go forth, and stand upon the mount before the LORD. And, behold, the LORD passed by, and a great and strong wind rent the mountains, and brake in pieces the rocks before the LORD; but the LORD was not in the wind: and after the wind an earthquake; but the LORD was not in the earthquake: 12 And after the earthquake a fire; but the LORD was not in the fire: and after the fire a still small voice.

He speaks to us in many ways, but they all have one thing in common – we have to be listening.

I have to laugh about what I am about to say; it brings to mind when people hear the story I just related. Without fail, they say that he was lucky. I respond by saying, "Lucky is the day the tractor does not run over you." Our family has been truly blessed; dad has survived cancer, heart attack, stroke, and being run over by a tractor. Mom has fought cancer and lung problems stemming from the treatment; both are approaching ninety years of age. Barbie has come through her battle better than could have been hoped for. These were times when the Lord spoke loudly.

I also think of the times that he has brought us through the dangers that we never saw – the days when one route to town was chosen over another, seemingly for no reason, the many small day to day decisions that go unnoticed. What could a different decision have led us into?

I think of the story of the old preacher back in the days of travel by horse. He pastored a church at the end of a long narrow ridge only accessible by a narrow path going up a steep hill. A young visiting preacher filled in while the old pastor took a trip. Upon his return, he asked the young preacher how things had went. The young preacher excitedly told him of the night his horse had run off on him, as they went down the hill. He told him how the Lord had preserved his life that night. The old preacher said, "Yes the Lord has saved my life on that hill many times." The young preacher asked, "Did your horse run off on you too?" The old preacher replied, "No, the Lord never let him."

How often the Lord never lets hardship or trouble come to us we may never know. But we should be thankful, even when one gets through.

Through the years, I have taken many decisions to the Lord, some are answered by doors being swung wide open;

leaving no doubt as to what is the right decision. Not real long after I got back into church, the preacher said someone would need to take on the role of adult Sunday school teacher. I prayed about it and decided to give it a try; I am far into the second trip through the Bible now, each takes about ten years. Looking back it has benefited me in my career also, as I am often called upon to teach in our yearly trainings. I have had job decisions to make when the only thing I heard was an uneasiness about the decision I was about to make. A couple of times I have turned down better offers to go where if felt I had peace in the decision. Again hindsight has confirmed the correct decision was made.

Isa 30:21 And thine ears shall hear a word behind thee, saying, This is the way, walk ye in it, when ye turn to the right hand, and when ye turn to the left.

Yes, the guidance is there, but the listening is the hard part, as we go through life many decisions are made without thought, much less prayer. Each small decision we make in life can and will alter the path we are on, each should be made carefully. I do not give this advice as one who always follows it, but as one who wishes he did.

I think often of Barbie hearing the simple words "go on." This has guided her in several big decisions. When she hears this she does not waiver, but charges headlong into the situation. Be it going forward to salvation, brain surgery, radiation or chemo. He seems to speak louder to her, but she listens. I often ask her to pray about our life decisions and listen to her response eagerly. It is great when she has the same feeling or answer that I do. He speaks in many ways if we are listening. My brother, after spending three or four days at various hospitals with his newborn grandson, who was born with serious health issues, and after many days praying for strength and help. He walked into a gift shop in a daze that comes from those situations, spun a greeting card rack around stood face to face with a card that spoke directly to his prayers.

He speaks to us to answer our prayers, to comfort us and to call us to salvation, His voice is everywhere, it's our choice to listen or not.

Ro 1:19 Because that which may be known of God is manifest in them; for God hath shewed it unto them.

20 For the invisible things of him from the creation of the world are clearly seen, being understood by the things that are made, even his eternal power and Godhead; so that they are without excuse:

Prayer has been such an important part of our journey, one that would have been very hard to do without. Many times I have found myself lying awake in bed, things from the day or things ahead of us, worry keeping me from sleep. I have talked to the Lord about them, acknowledged that they are in His power and that I trust him for the outcome. Then I roll over and go to sleep. Had I not of had that option, I would have worried all night, and to many of those nights take a toll on a person. Again His voice is there, speaking peace that allows a good night's sleep. Many times His voice is heard in the outcome, the prayer answered, and the peace that is there even when things do not go as we wish.

We often hear it said that everything happens for a reason, and I believe it does. Then we hear that one day we will know all about it. I do not know if I believe that, I think that when we get out of this life, the things that have happened will not be important anymore. When I have reached the afterlife, I will not want to revisit all the things that have saddened me in this life. I will not care about them but only about the paradise surrounding me.

I have talked about many prayers answered in a way that I rejoiced in, but I have had many that the answer was not what I wanted to hear. The story I have been telling is heavy with results that are not what I prayed for. These prayers were also answered, but not the way I wanted. We should always remember that He knows what is best, and often it is not what we are praying for.

Isa 55:8 For my thoughts are not your thoughts, neither are your ways my ways, saith the LORD.

9 For as the heavens are higher than the earth, so are my ways higher than your ways, and my thoughts than your thoughts.

10 For as the rain cometh down, and the snow from heaven, and returneth not thither, but watereth the earth, and maketh it bring forth and bud, that it may give seed to the sower, and bread to the eater:

11 So shall my word be that goeth forth out of my mouth: it shall not return unto me void, but it shall accomplish that which I please, and it shall prosper in the thing whereto I sent it.

The prayers that are not answered the way we want are the answers that are harder to hear and to understand. For me, many times I find that years later I can see there was an answer, and it was the best. At first, all I saw was things going terribly wrong, these are the times when we had to rely on our faith. We had to trust in him and ask for his will to be done, and accept that it may not be our will. But it has been my experience that he is faithful.

Heb 10:23 Let us hold fast the profession of our faith without wavering; (for he is faithful that promised;)

I our sincere hope is that we have helped someone who is in a dark place, who has taken the plunge into darkness, and it seems that all hope is far away.

Not
The End

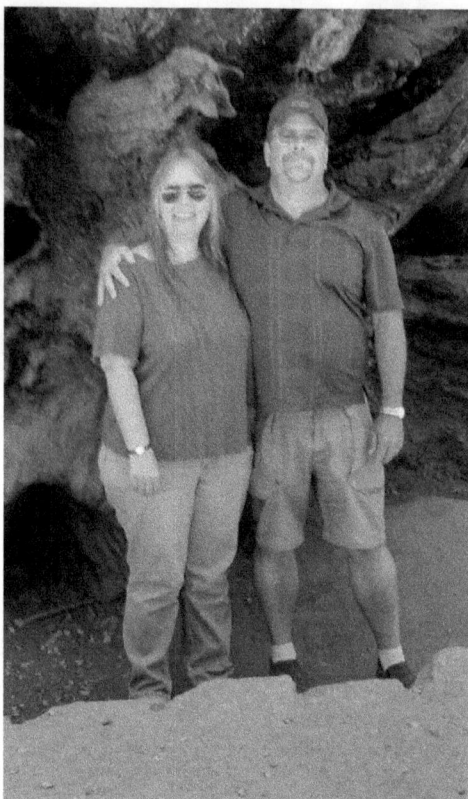

Barbie and Dave Renfroe

ABOUT THE AUTHORS

DAVE RENFROE is a long-time owner of a family farm and a claims manager for a crop insurance company. Since August 1999, Dave's spouse Barbie has suffered from brian cancer, and he served as her caretaker during much of that time. BARBIE RENFROE has worked as a farmer and homemaker but is currently engaged in her fight full time. The Renfroes reside in Lawrence County, Ohio. You can learn more about Barbie's struggle at *davebarbierenfroe.com.*

www.ingramcontent.com/pod-product-compliance
Lightning Source LLC
LaVergne TN
LVHW021503080426
835509LV00018B/2384